There Is a Cure

for Arthritis

There <u>Is</u> a Cure

for Arthritis

by

Paavo O. Airola, N.D.

PARKER PUBLISHING COMPANY, INC.
WEST NYACK, NEW YORK

This book is a reference work based on research by
the author. The opinions expressed herein are not
necessarily those of or endorsed by the publisher.
The directions stated in this book are in no way
to be considered as a substitute for consultation
with a duly licensed doctor.

ISBN 0-13-914671-7 PBK

ISBN 0-13-914698-9 RWD CLASSIC PBK

Dedicated to the practitioners of the healing arts who have the unprejudiced and inquiring minds to search for the truth and, when found, the courage to proclaim it and use it for the benefit of their patients—even if the truth happens to be contrary to the accepted orthodox thinking and practices.

A Foreword by a Doctor of Medicine

Modern medicine is in a state of dilemma. On one hand, technological development is accelerated to an unprecedented tempo. Chemistry and the physical-technological sciences have totally captured all fields of therapy. On the other hand, this trend is simultaneously accompanied by the catastrophic increase of the chronic degenerative diseases.

Many of our time's most responsible and visionary researchers have suggested a possible causative connection between these two trends. They have appealed for moderation and thoughtfulness. Can chemical substances adequately and harmlessly replace the biological processes? Are pharmacological conclusions drawn from animal experiments applicable and relevant in a human clinic? Modern toxicology and the recent mass tragedies connected with the use of drugs suggest that the above question can not be answered in the affirmative.

The catastrophic point of no return to which chemically and technologically oriented medicine has evolved, has given basis for new medical thinking: biological medicine. Its assertion is that the physical-chemical laws can not be indiscriminately applied on the biological reality, with its multiplicity of distinctive and unique characteristics, without assaulting the objective criteria of the reality one is trying to serve. The biological phenomena are not subordinated to the physical-chemical laws—

they are, on the contrary, superior to them. While conventional, orthodox medicine considers that chemical substances can substitute for the biological processes, biological medicine rejects such thinking as a form of modern superstition. The biological processes can only be understood in their unique peculiarity. The pathological abnormalities in the biological processes can only be corrected by changes in the biological environment. Bacteria or virus are not primary causes of disease; they are only symptomatic factors of the biological milieu. To correct this milieu is of the utmost importance for the successful management of disease. Chemical drugs can, at their best, serve only for the temporary relief of symptoms. Prolonged use of drugs will always damage the biological milieu. The normalizing of this milieu, or creating of the biological environment most conducive for the healing processes, is the prime goal of the biologically oriented physician.

Many patients have been restored to health through the practiced application of biological medicine after all the conventional treatments have failed. Biological medicine and naturopathic methods of treatment will come to the fore more and more as the successful alternative to conventional therapy; and for the afflicted, who tried in vain conventional therapy, they present the only choice. The philosophy of biological medicine is not in opposition to conventional medicine; it rather widens, deepens and complements it.

From the rich flora of degenerative diseases of modern civilized man the author of this book has chosen rheumatoid arthritis to test the effectiveness of biological medicine. It is common knowledge that the conventional therapies are unable to help arthritis sufferers, as far as permanent results are concerned, with the possible exception of temporary relief of the symptoms. The author has made an objective analysis of biological therapeutic treatments applied in the management of arthritis and the results obtained.

It is to be hoped that this competent, instructive and inspiring book could aid in the downfall of established dogma, promulgated by orthodox medicine, that "there is no cure for arthritis." If this preconceived tenet can be disproved, would it not give reason to assume that the same is true with others of our most common degenerative diseases? From the basis of rheumatoid arthritis this book shows the incompatibility of such a dogmatic conventional attitude. If the author can help to tear down the high prison-walls of preconceived ideas, which prevent us from seeing the sun-drenched views of glorious health —and thus stimulate interest for biological medicine—then he has accomplished a great service for disease-ridden mankind.

However, a word of caution should be expressed. Just as it is bad to be caught in the vicious cycle of prejudiced conventional and preconceived ideas, it is equally foolish to adopt an inane optimism which is out of touch with realities. We must judge the possibilities offered by biological medicine realistically and acknowledge its limitations. These are in direct relationship with the body's own restorative capacities. Where the damage effected by the prolonged therapy with chemical drugs and corticosteroids is so extensive that it had caused the glandular atrophy and the impairment in the body's own healing mechanism, or where there are extensive degenerative changes in the joints, then even biological medicine will be but of little help.

Nevertheless, after reading this book, one must draw the conclusion that every passing year, that conventional medicine, wrapped in prejudiced thinking, is unwilling to change its attitude and thinking pattern and ignores the existence of biological medicine, a countless number of people will be subjected to needless and prolonged suffering.

LARS-ERIK ESSÉN, M.D.

Acknowledgments

I wish to express my sincere thanks and indebtedness to the following persons for their unselfish contribution and assistance in assembling the material for this book and/or proofreading it before publication:

KARL-OTTO ALY, M.D.
LARS-ERIK ESSÉN, M.D.
JERN HAMBERG, M.D.
WILLIAM M. McGAREY, M.D.
C. A. CALL, D.C., N.D.
MRS. ALMA NISSEN
MRS. INGRID ÖYE-CARLSON

I am particularly indebted to Drs. William M. McGarey, M.D., and Lars-Erik Essén, M.D. for proofreading the manuscript and for their valuable advice which resulted in many pertinent changes in the content and presentation of the subject.

My special thanks to the editors of Swedish Magazine *Tidskrift för Hälsa*, Mr. Eskil Svensson and Mr. Arne Algard, for their cooperation and kindness in granting permission to use material from the magazine in this book. Chapters 2, 3, 13, and 16 are in part based on the articles published in *Tidskrift för Hälsa*.

I also wish to express my sincere thanks to Mrs. Pat Jarvis and Mrs. Marsha Merwin for their linguistic assistance in preparation of this book—help as much appreciated as it was needed.

INTRODUCTION

It is estimated that over 13 million Americans are afflicted with arthritis in its various forms. Arthritis is, perhaps, the most crippling and agonizing of all degenerative diseases. Although not as great a direct killer as, for example, cancer and heart diseases, arthritis causes more pain, despair, and suffering to more people than any other single disease.

The most distressing fact about arthritis is that 13 million or more arthritis sufferers are given no hope for cure or even any relief from their discomfort and misery. At regular intervals new drugs will pop up on the market, hailed as long-sought miracle remedies, lighting momentarily a spark of new hope and anticipation in the millions of distressed minds reaching for a last straw. But eventually they all turn out to be cruel disappointments. Sulfa drugs, aspirin, gold injections, cortisone, ACTH—all have proven to be failures as far as permanent results in arthritis are concerned.

An announcement of the discovery of cortisone was met with great joy and excitement by doctors and arthritis sufferers. Crippled patients would be able to walk, stiff joints would become mobile and pain-free as if by magic. To millions of people with arthritis around the world cortisone held out the great promise that at last an effective remedy for the disease had been found. But the exalted enthusiasm was promptly replaced by cruel disappointment! It soon became evident that "the remedy was worse than the disease." Cortisone has caused so many toxic reactions and dangerous side effects that it is now considered "on the way out" in the treatment of arthritis.

Meanwhile, millions of disillusioned arthritis sufferers are left without hope with their agonizing pain and misery. They have nowhere to turn for help. After trying all the existing orthodox treatments and drugs, which did not give them any lasting help, they are at a complete loss as to what to try next. "Official" medicine and the Arthritis Foundation assure them that there is no cure for arthritis. Millions of dollars are collected yearly for research aimed at discovery of a drug which will be able to cure arthritis. It is evident, however, that we are doomed to new disappointments. Arthritis is a systemic, metabolic disease, the end result of a longtime abuse of normal bodily processes, and cannot be expected to be cured by a single miracle drug. Only by correcting and eliminating the underlying causes and abnormal conditions which caused its development can arthritis be successfully corrected.

While medicine at large is in the dark concerning causes and effective treatments for arthritis, biologically oriented medical doctors and naturopathic practitioners, both in the United States and Europe, have developed biological methods of treatment which have proven to be most successful in healing many diseases, including arthritis.

This book brings arthritis sufferers good news.

Inspired by enthusiastic reports from many European clinics on biological therapies for arthritis, I have recently made several visits to Europe to study firsthand these biological methods and the results attained through them. In sharp contrast to the situation in this country where biological medicine is virtually nonexistent, in Europe it is a fast growing branch of medical science. Hundreds of biologically oriented medical doctors are researching and developing new biological therapies and applying them on most, if not all, existing plagues of mankind. In Sweden, Germany, Switzerland, England, and Finland you can find dozens of clinics operated by medical doctors or naturopathic practitioners who specialize in biological methods of treatment.

I have visited many of these clinics. I have interviewed many doctors and hundreds of patients. I have checked and studied the records of the case histories of these patients. I have seen with my own eyes how patients with arthritis, crippled for years, have left their crutches and beds and walked. Many patients with tears of joy in their eyes told me of their wonderful experiences at the biological clinics. After a few days or weeks of simple and harmless treatments, the pain from which they suffered for years disappeared and their joints became mobile and flexible again.

This book is written with the sole aim of bringing good news of these successful biological treatments to millions of arthritis sufferers and freeing them from their hopelessness and desperation. My happy message to them is that they should not despair. Biological medicine has an answer to their problem. In the following chapters I will report on many actual cases with detailed descriptions of their case histories and all the treatments employed which led to their complete cure. I will also outline a program of biological methods, based on the experience of European clinics but adapted to American conditions, which could be successfully applied by arthritis sufferers in their own homes or under supervision of their own physicians.

I wish to stress the fact that this book does not promulgate my own theories, hypotheses, and conclusions. I do not prescribe nor do I advance a new cure for arthritis.

My mission is that of an objective reporter presenting the facts—as I have found them—for your consideration. Biological medicine is not quackery nor a passing new fad. It is a true medical science based on the principle of intelligent support of the natural healing power inherent in the living organism. Biological medicine is based on the teachings of the great Hippocrates, the "Father of Medicine," that no drugs ever cure disease. Lasting results can be attained only when a wise doctor assists and supports the body's own healing forces, which institute the health-restoring processes and accomplish the actual cure. Biological treatments are directed at correcting underlying causes of the disease, strengthening the patient's resistance, and creating the most favorable conditions for these healing processes to take place. Hundreds of licensed medical practitioners in Europe use the biological therapies outlined in this book in treating their patients.

It is my conviction that if you read this book with an open and unprejudiced mind and follow the outlined programs, you will soon be convinced that biological medicine is as scientific as it is "common sense," and that the sufferers of this crippling disease need not despair—*there is*, indeed, a *cure for arthritis!*

Paavo O. Airola, N.D.

An Appeal to the Members of the Medical Profession

Profound changes are taking place in medical thinking. The era of specialization and the tendency to see man as a chemo-physical conglomeration of many separate parts is giving place to a new biological thinking. This new school of thought is directed towards the concept of man as a whole person with his physical, emotional, and spiritual aspects inseparably unified in one living soul. The place of man as an organic part of the biological and cosmic universe, subject to all the unchangeable and irrevocable laws of nature, is increasingly recognized.

The role of nutrition in preventive and therapeutic medicine has become increasingly evident. Biochemical imbalance due to faulty dietary patterns is recognized as the major causative factor in many chronic and degenerative diseases of civilized man. Recent findings point to nutritional and environmental factors as leading culprits in the general deterioration of health and the alarming increase in degenerative diseases. It becomes increasingly evident that the present-day conventional drug approach is unable to solve the problem of catastrophic increases of such diseases as cancer, cardiovascular disorders, diabetes, arthritis, etc. A more fundamental approach which takes man's environmental factors, nutritional patterns, and emotional attitudes into consideration is long overdue.

It is the responsibility and duty of all those who are engaged in the professions of healing and who are motivated by high standards of idealism and service to familiarize themselves with the newest developments in medical thinking, as well as the latest pertinent biochemical and nutritional facts, and utilize this knowledge in the management and instruction of their patients.

Presently, arthritis is a major threat to the health of this nation. It exceeds all other diseases in terms of human suffering and privation.

Arthritis has long been a "stepchild of medicine." Generally, medicine has admitted its complete inability to penetrate the mysteries and arrest the epidemic growth of this "foremost crippler" in the United States. Crippled and disabled arthritis sufferers, wracked with pain and disillusioned by the inability of orthodox doctors to give them help, often turn to quacks. It is estimated that over $250 million is wasted by arthritics yearly on falsely advertised or misrepresented products, gadgets, or quick cures. The recent (April, 1966) *Review of the Surgeon General's Workshop on the Prevention of Disability from Arthritis* stated: "Frequently, quackery flourishes because the physician who first sees the arthritis patient is not trained to cope adequately with the problem." As Dr. Cornelius Traeger, M.D., in the *Review of the Surgeon General's Workshop*, puts it, "The public is discouraged by lack of knowledge of arthritis and lack of interest when they visit the doctor. The public is confused by the lack of agreement among doctors with respect to various types of therapy." The report called for healing professions and scientific forces to make a united, all-out effort to eradicate this "major health hazard," which incapacitates 13 million Americans and costs the nation's economy about $2 billion a year.

The typical and very significant gap n the above-mentioned report, as well as in similar reports by the National Arthritis Foundation and the National Institute of Arthritis and Metabolic Diseases, is the conspicuous omission of the possible role of nutrition in the total picture of development and management of arthritis. Moreover, these official and federal arthritis research agencies are seemingly unaware of the many medical practitioners and researchers who are working on the development of biological arthritis therapies as a positive, promising alternative to the unsuccessful conventional drug approach.

It is difficult to believe that this ignorance is not self-imposed. There is an International Center for Biological Research in Europe with hundreds of doctors, scientists, and correspondents from all over the world, including the United States, participating as active members. There are many scientific publications and journals representing the views of biological medicine which publish the results of steadily growing research in this field. Dozens of clinics in Europe employ biological therapies under the direction of licensed physicians with extraordinary results.

European medical thinking is fast moving toward the new biological era of medical science, based on the philosophy that most diseases are of man's own making and are the result of health-destroying living habits, wrong nutritional patterns, and other harmful environmental factors. American "official" medicine and governmental health organizations continue to cling to an outdated medical philosophy based on the Pasteurian assumption that all diseases are caused by bacteria. Consequently, the main effort of present medical research is aimed at identifying the bacteria considered pathogenic and developing specific drugs to destroy the suspected bacteria. This conservative, rather old-fashioned thinking is perhaps to blame for the fact that research in many vital fields, including arthritis, has been so unsuccessful.

It is evident that the conventional symptomatic drug approach, including corticosteroid therapies, has sadly failed to show positive results in management of arthritis, and the whole present-day, orthodox approach to the disease is colored by hopelessness and uncertainty. A time is long overdue to completely re-evaluate conventional thinking and consider a return to the fundamental Hippocratic nature-cure principles, as promulgated by biological medicine.

It is my sincere hope that members of the medical profession who are motivated by high ideals of professional integrity and a sincere desire to serve their patients will avail themselves of the information presented in this book. They will then be able to better serve the needs of their patients and be of real help to arthritis sufferers.

Although this work is aimed at the average layman reader, the general philosophy of biological medicine and the descriptions of the suggested therapies are sufficiently comprehensive to give members of the medical profession necessary guidance in practical application of the recommended measures.

I appeal to all those with unprejudiced and inquiring minds, who search for the truth, to examine the biological common-sense approach to arthritis and give it an objective, unbiased test. It is natural to be doubtful, even skeptical, when confronted with something which is new and unorthodox. But let the results be the determining factor as to which approach is more effective. After all, in medicine there is only one criterion for the value of any given remedy: Does it work? If the remedy works, if the therapy can bring about permanent betterment or cure—then it is the correct one, even if it happens to be contrary to accepted thinking and endorsed conventional practices!

We should never forget that medical history is full of persistent intolerance, even violent opposition, by orthodox practitioners to new unorthodox philosophies and unconventional healing methods. Virtually every major medical discovery was met with antagonism and organized opposition. The stories of Lord Lister, Ignaz Semmelweis, Szent-Györgyi, Louis Pasteur, Mesmer, and presently Drs. Shutes, Max Gerson, and Andrew C. Ivy are just a few striking examples of the fierce opposition, ridicule, and persecution which await anyone who dares to make a major medical discovery or support it!

It has been said that every new idea is blankly rejected, suppressed, and ridiculed by the contemporary generation; openly discussed and evaluated by the following generation; and, finally, gratefully accepted, endorsed, and incorporated to the general practice by the third generation.

Biological medicine is in its first generation! Do not wait for two generations to reap the benefits of the extraordinary values it can add to your arsenal of therapeutic measures.

Biological medicine is not opposed to any of the healing systems, including the medical. Rather it complements them. Its philosophy is based on the fundamental principle of intelligent cooperation with nature; it sees man as a part of nature, subject to its eternal laws. It is a modern science which incorporates all the harmless and effective therapies that can be applied in the correction of disease and restoration of health.

It is my sincere hope that conscientious medical men will permit nothing to stand in their way in applying these most effective therapies—even if they are new and unconventional. As R. P. Watterson, M.D. said: "Although not in general use, knowledge of the cause of arthritis exists as well as measures necessary for its prevention and treatment. It is the obligation of the medical profession to recognize and use this information." *

Arthritis sufferers are crying for help. They deserve all the help they can get. They are looking up to you for the alleviation of their agonizing existence. The *Surgeon General's Report on Arthritis* called for a concerted effort of all concerned to eradicate arthritis, this "foremost crippler, by all available means." Don't let complacency, indifference, and medical prejudice stand in the way of progress! Let the welfare of your patients be your *only* consideration. Practice your great mission and call with this noble goal in mind. An open-minded study of material presented in this book will help you achieve this goal and "break the arthritic's frustrating chain of hopelessness."

Paavo O. Airola, N.D.

* R. P. Watterson, M.D. "Arthritis: Biochemical Suffocation," *Southwestern Medicine,* Vol. 42, No. 4, April, 1961.

Contents

Part One

THERE
IS
A CURE!

Chapter 1

The "Miracles" at Brandal

My first confrontation with biological methods of treatment for arthritis was at Brandals Health Clinic located in Södertälje, a little idyllic suburb town, a few miles south of Stockholm, Sweden.

Alma Nissen, directress of the Brandals Clinic, met me at the railway station. For the past 12 years I have followed the work of Alma Nissen through the Swedish magazine *Tidskrift för Hälsa* (the *Magazine for Health*) which has published many remarkable cases of arthritis cures accomplished at Brandal. Mrs. Nissen, after curing her own arthritis a few decades ago, has dedicated her whole life to helping thousands of other arthritis sufferers.

A fortyish-looking, dark-blonde, slim, elegant lady stepped from her station wagon, warmly greeted me with "Välkommen," opened the back door, and threw my heavy bags in. Then she walked around the car and opened the door for me, which made me feel rather old at 50. Imagine my surprise when I found that

3

she is 70! And not a grey hair on her head! There was no doubt
in my mind that whatever her "method" is, it certainly works
for her!

The Brandals Clinic is beautifully located on the shore of
the Baltic Sea and is surrounded by majestic woods. An ideal
natural setting for rest and contemplation with a "back-to-
nature" atmosphere. It is an old three-floor villa with a huge
sitting room featuring a TV, grand piano, other musical instru-
ments, library, and a collection of crutches and prostheses left
here by grateful patients who didn't need them any more.
The clinic has facilities for accommodation and treatment of
30 patients. At the time of my visit—July, 1966—it was filled to
capacity.

Alma Nissen's Own Story

"Tell me, how and why did you become interested in arthritis
and what prompted you to open this clinic?" This was my first
question when we met at a smorgasbord table in the dining
room at Brandal.

"Twenty-five years ago I was so incapacitated by arthritis
that I was practically bedridden. After trying all the available
medical treatments, consulting dozens of doctors, and several
fruitless stays in hospitals I was becoming progressively worse.
My hands and fingers were stiff and in constant pain. I could
not bend myself, walk, or even turn myself in bed. In addition, I
had a chronic ovary inflammation and constant migraine. I was
suffering from a bad case of insomnia with resulting nervous
exhaustion. I also was chronically constipated...

"I felt hopeless. Nobody could help me. I could not see my
way out of the indescribable suffering I had to endure. But my
spirit was strong and wouldn't give up. I was not willing to
accept my lot as a bedridden invalid for the rest of my life.
With the typical Scandinavian *sisu* and perseverance I rebelled
against my fate. I wanted to live, become healthy again...

"A book by a British physician, Sir Robert McCarrison, gave me new hope and become the turning point in my life. It opened my eyes to the relation between nutrition and health. I started to experiment with myself. I changed my diet. I fasted. I drank fresh vegetable juices and broths made with cooked vegetables. I drank herb teas. I took enemas and utilized colonic irrigation to cleanse my intestines of accumulated toxins and wastes. I read all I could on the nature-cure methods and picked up ideas here and there. I met the famous Danish raw-diet pioneer Dr. Kristine Nolfi, M.D., and read and studied her book *The Living Foods*. I also took heat treatments and hydro-baths. I must admit, I didn't have faith in much of what I did, but desperate as I was, I was willing to try anything.

"Imagine my surprise, when I started to feel better and better! The stiffness in my joints started to disappear. I slept better; pain gave way, and after just a few months I was, to my and everybody's amazement, completely cured!

"This was 25 years ago and I never had a sick day since. No traces of arthritis...Would you like to see how flexible and elastic my body is?"

With this she took her shoes off and gave me a gymnastic demonstration which many a young athlete would be proud to equal.

"But I do have visible evidence of my former arthritis. The toes on my feet were so deformed and the joints so fused together, that they never have straightened out completely. Look at them!

"When damage is so extensive that joints are completely destroyed and fused together, nothing can restore them, not even biological methods. But in the great majority of cases, even with deformation, but of shorter duration, the complete restoration of health is possible.

"Now, when I cured myself I was so overjoyed with the discoveries I made that I wanted to share them with others and help as many as I could. I visited Dr. McCarrison and he advised me to open a clinic and help other arthritics regain their health.

"Encouraged by the enthusiastic endorsement of this great scientist, I transformed my seven-room apartment in Copenhagen to an arthritis clinic. Patients came from everywhere. They were brought in on stretchers; they came supported on crutches; they came in wheelchairs. And after four to eight weeks on my simple regime they left the clinic on their own feet, without wheelchairs and crutches. The grateful patients spread the news of their cures and a long line of patients were waiting to come in under my care.

"My arthritis therapies and extraordinary results became widely publicized in the press. The Norwegian Medical Association invited me to present a lecture on my therapies before the leading medical authorities of the country and the students of the Oslo Medical School. Well-known rheumatologists such as Prof. Olav Hanssen, Dr. V. G. Kofoed, Professor Roald Opsaht and others attended and took part in the discussions.

"My fame spread to Sweden and a wealthy benefactor offered the Brandal, a beautiful estate with a large villa, for my disposition, to be used as a rheumatic clinic. I accepted gratefully. That was 13 years ago. During these years we have helped thousands of arthritis sufferers . . ."

My First Day at Brandal

My first day at Brandal was mostly spent walking in the huge, shady woods, which surround the estate, and listening to Mrs. Nissen tell of her work.

At 5:00 P.M. the bell rang and called all for dinner. I found about half of the patients in the living room, the other half in the dining room. Those in the living room were the "fasting" patients, who were served fruit juice or vegetable broth.

I joined the "eating" patients in the adjoining dining room, where the huge, festive table, decorated with flowers and candles, was filled with colorful and delicious lactovegetarian courses. It was a smorgasbord at its best! The table was laden with at least ten kinds of different salads of fresh, organically grown vegetables; cottage cheese with cummin; baked potatoes, sauerkraut, tomato soup, soybean purée, buttermilk, whey cheese, whole grain bread, and fresh butter. Some guests, just off fast, were advised to avoid certain dishes, mostly bread and cooked foods, but others, including yours truly, enjoyed the whole colorful palette of appetizing "råkost."

After dinner everyone assembled in the living room—*Salongen* —to watch TV. The favorite Swedish show, *10,000 Crown Question,* was on and everyone sat in a state of hypnotized attention waiting for the answers of the competing "experts." It reminded me of our TV in the mid-fifties and the famed scandals of the *$64,000 Question.*

When the *10,000 Crown Question* was followed by the *Andy Williams Show,* that was enough for me, and I left the *Salongen* for my room and a good night's sleep.

The "Miracles"

The next morning developments followed in a fast tempo, which prompted me to use the word "miracle" in the subtitle above.

A little Danish woman, who had depended on her crutches for years, left them behind and walked through the hall outside of my room without them. This was her eighth fasting day. She never needed the crutches again.

Another lady from Gothenburg reported that the pain in her joints disappeared on the second day of her fast and that on the fourth day she was able to leave her crutches.

On a big, sunny balcony I met several patients trying to catch as much as they could of the warm, life-giving sun—in a country where sun is so scarce.

A young girl of approximately 20, was rolled onto the balcony

in a wheelchair. She had been afflicted with arthritis for seven
years and was a complete invalid. Her hands were grotesquely
deformed. She could not move or lift her legs. She came to
Brandal in a wheelchair and was still in a wheelchair. But she
was already feeling much better, her pain was gone. She was
determined to continue fasting for a few more weeks in the
hope that she might leave her wheelchair there.

I also met a 43-year-old woman from Stockholm. She had
been ill with arthritis for 14 years. For 14 long years she visited
hospital after hospital, took drug after drug. You name it—
she'd had it: gold injection, cortisone, Imagon, Butazolidin,
etc. The best arthritis specialists in the country from Söder-
sjukhuset and the famous Karolinska Institute in Stockholm
treated her until finally they all gave up, admitting that they
could do nothing more. She had come to the clinic just five
days before and started fasting immediately.

"I am so happy. It is unbelievable!" she said to me with enthusiasm. "In just four days all pain is gone. I could not
straighten this leg before—look at it now! It is completely
straight. After 14 years of pain and suffering—it is just unbelievable! It's a miracle!"

As I walked on the balcony among all these sunbathing men
and women, this word "miracle" lingered in my mind. In this
clinic alone—and the little country of Sweden has at least half
a dozen other clinics with similar biological methods of treatment—thousands of hopeless arthritis sufferers were helped;
most of them to a complete recovery. Crippled, deformed,
doomed to lifelong invalidism, labeled by official medical authorities as incurable, they had come there as a last resort.
After a few weeks of simple biological treatments, without
fancy drugs and injections, they walked away happy and grateful, restored to complete health. Is this a miracle?

The Real Miracle!

Actually, there is no *miracle cure* for arthritis! As a matter of fact, there is no *specific,* singular curative therapy for arthritis. No specific treatment, no specific diet, no specific bath possesses curative properties which can cure arthritis. The cure is accomplished by the healing power inherent in the body itself. The biological treatments only release and actively support this healing power, creating the most favorable conditions for repair, rebuilding, and re-establishment of health.

As I studied the actual cases, interviewed the patients, and observed the various biological treatments used to bring about these remarkable recoveries, I could not help but think that the miracle is not in the fact that these patients are cured, but that these biological methods, which can accomplish such extraordinary results, and which are so widely used in Europe, are virtually unknown in the United States!

This to me is a real miracle: *That millions of arthritis sufferers in the U.S.A., hopeless and disillusioned in their despair, have never heard that such methods exist.* They are in complete ignorance of the great developments which are now taking place in biological medicine.

It is a miracle, indeed, that the biological methods described in this book are unknown to the public in this country and that 13 million American arthritis sufferers are pacified by repeated, paid commercials which say, "There is no cure for arthritis"!

Chapter 2

He Left His Crutches and Walked

Albin Vistrand, 60, a Swedish farmer from Bie, Sörmland, suffered from agonizing arthritis for 12 years.[1]

Actually it all started long ago. While in military service during his youth he hurt his right arm. The infection spread and developed into a bad blood poisoning. After the operation his arm didn't heal completely and he was discharged as an invalid. For several years he was bothered with open, inflamed ulcers until the arm was finally healed. Then for many years he enjoyed seemingly perfect health.

But in 1953 the same arm was stricken with a severe attack of arthritis. Not only was he unable to perform his farm labors, but he could not write, not even peel his potatoes. After two years of suffering and pain he was finally ordered by doctors to use a prosthesis on his arm to enable him to bend it at all.

[1] From *Tidskrift för Hälsa,* January, 1966. Used by permission.

He had this prosthesis on his arm every day for ten long years!

In 1957 arthritis started to spread to other parts of the body. His left leg became badly inflamed. Increasing stiffness accompanied the unbearable pain. He also received a bigger prosthesis for his leg, which limited his movements and made walking with crutches more bearable.

In addition to various drugs, one doctor gave instructions to wrap the leg in adhesive bandage.

"This treatment I'll never forget," said Mr. Vistrand.

The bandage was left on for several weeks and, finally, when the pain became so bad that he could not stand it anymore, he called the doctor. "Try to remove the bandage," was the doctor's advice.

"I did," continued Mr. Vistrand. "I worked for two hours with a pair of scissors and a razor blade, and when I finished the whole leg looked like bloody flesh and pus."

Now he started the long list of visits to various hospitals and arthritis clinics. Eight weeks in Kullbergska Hospital ... Three weeks in Norrtuna Hospital ... without any improvement in his condition. In Eskilstuna Hospital he received 12 x-ray treatments for his left knee. After this treatment the knee was so badly burned that they had to operate on it. In addition, he was stricken by double pneumonia. When he finally came back home, his arthritis was worse than ever.

"I had such frightful pains that it is impossible to describe them," he said.

Now some friends recommended the well-known cure clinic for rheumatic diseases in Nynäshamn. Mr. Vistrand went there in November, 1958 and stayed until the end of January, 1959. Treatments consisted of various forms of physiotherapy, baths, and massage, plus masses of different drugs. He felt a little better and the drugs killed the pain. When he returned home, however, his pain came back.

The next hospital visit was to Löt. Here the entire treatment consisted of various drugs—14 tablets each day. It was in this hospital that his leg prosthesis of steel and leather was made in an attempt to hold his leg in a straight position.

In spite of all these various treatments and drugs, his condition was getting progressively worse. Now both his legs were affected. A visit to a famous rheumatologist at St. Erik's Hospital in Stockholm, revealed that he also was afflicted with a bad anemia due to an iron deficiency. He received 20 injections of iron in addition to several new drugs, including Butazolidin. They helped to relieve the pain, but now he was seized with cramps in the legs and his toenails turned black and fell off. But his blood quality improved and he started to gain weight.

Then his heart started to bother him. A new visit to a doctor resulted in a new drug for his heart condition. He discovered, however, that when he took his heart medicine, it completely disrupted his stomach and digestion. And when he took his drugs for arthritis they affected his heart condition—the typical vicious cycle of drug therapy!

He began to realize that he was at the end of his rope. In his search for relief he had tried everything and nothing had helped. His arthritis was becoming worse with each week. He took 22 tablets of various drugs each day, but they didn't give him any lasting relief. He felt desperate, helpless, and discouraged.

It was at that time that some friends showed him a copy of *Tidskrift för Hälsa* which opened his eyes to an alternative to drugs and operations—a new biological approach to the treatment of arthritis. One cold and dark day in January, 1964 he was taken in an automobile to the Brandals Clinic.

"I was very skeptical when I arrived there," he says. "After all, I went through so many different treatments before, without getting better. Also, I was instructed to get rid of all tablets and my program should start with an enema and potato broth—a water in which potatoes were boiled!"

Twenty-Five Days without Food

His program of treatments at Brandal started with a thera·
peutic fast which lasted 25 days. He received no solid foods,
only vegetable and fruit juices, vegetable broths, and herb teas.
His other treatments included alternating hot and cold showers
each morning, an enema twice a day, colonic irrigation once a
week, exercises, and lots of rest.

After 20 days of fasting he was able to leave his crutches
and walk without them. On the 26th day he started eating
again. His diet consisted of raw fruits and vegetables with
homemade yogurt, wheat germ, crushed seeds and nuts, vege·
table soup, and potatoes.

One week after completion of the fast he was able to climb
the stairs to the second floor without help and without even
holding onto the handrail. The pain had disappeared com·
pletely. He had full mobility of his arms and legs.

Mr. Vistrand wrapped his arm and leg prostheses in a pack·
age and presented them to Alma Nissen as a new addition to
her "museum." They are proudly exhibited in the sitting room
of the Brandals Clinic for the inspiration of other arthritis
sufferers who come there.

Happy and optimistic Albin Vistrand returned to his farm
able to walk and work without crutches, without pain, and
without drugs. As a pleasant bonus from the biological thera·
pies at Brandal his heart and stomach problems disappeared
as well.

Chapter 3

Kajsa Andersson's Lasting Cure

Life had been good to Mrs. Kajsa Andersson, from Smål-andstenar, Sweden.[1] Five healthy and handsome children—happy family life—thriving small family business. All would have been rosy and sunny, but for one thing. After the last baby was born, Mrs. Andersson didn't seem to be able to recover her strength. She was always tired and listless. She could hardly lift up her arms. She lost her interest in everything, and just wanted to stay in bed and rest. Then came the pain in her arms and hands. A visit to a doctor and a dreadful diagnosis: rheumatoid arthritis!

The doctor prescribed a drug and ordered her to stay in bed with warm packs around the affected joints. Warm packs seemed to help relieve the pain, or rather to chase it to another joint. As soon as the hands felt better, the pain moved to the elbows. From the elbows it moved to the shoulders. Then her legs and feet started to ache, too. The drug relieved her pains

[1] From *Tidskrift för Hälsa*, May, 1962. Used by permission.

somewhat, but only for a short time. As soon as she was without the pills, the pains returned with increased strength.

After four weeks in bed with increasing disability and pain, which became more and more agonizing, she finally was remitted by her doctor to Spenshults Rheumatic Hospital, one of the most modern medical rheumatic clinics in Sweden. She stayed there six weeks. She didn't receive many treatments, except drugs and rest in bed, plus a typical hospital diet of plenty of meat, desserts, and coffee.

She felt a little better when she returned to her home. But as soon as she started to work around the house the stiffness and pain in the joints reappeared. She felt discouraged and hopeless, being unable to take care of her home and her children. All she had to look forward to was a dreadful future as a helpless invalid.

One day her nurse brought her a magazine with an article on the Brandals Clinic and biological medicine. After she had finished reading, she immediately went to the telephone and made a reservation.

She went to Brandal on October 20, 1957. That day she will never forget. She arrived there very sick and with agonizing pains. She could not get out of the taxi without help. She could not go up the stairs to her room. She could not dress nor undress herself. She was helpless and felt terrible pain with the slightest movement.

The program of treatments at Brandal started with the traditional fasting on vegetable broth and carrot juice. Among the other treatments were an alternating hot and cold shower, a dry brush massage, an enema in the morning and evening, and sleeping with the windows open while the scent of pinewood aroma filled her bedroom.

"After one week of fasting I felt so much better that I wanted to continue," she said. "And I continued as long as I felt that fasting was doing me good—for 20 days."

"After the first week I could go up and down the stairs and

take short walks outside. And every day my outdoor walks became longer and longer. I felt as if life was returning to me—a most wonderful feeling!"

After 20 days of fasting, one more week on the lactovegetarian diet, and other biological therapies at Brandal, Mrs. Andersson returned to her home—completely free from her arthritis, happy and full of hope for her and her family's healthy future.

This was in 1957. In 1962, five years after her phenomenal arthritis cure, she was interviewed by a correspondent from *Tidskrift för Hälsa* to determine the permanency of her cure.

"During these last five years I have not been sick a single day," said Mrs. Andersson. "I did not even have a cold or a running nose! The only reminder of arthritis I have is that if I work unusually long days using extremely hard labor, like washing clothes by hand or such, I feel a slight stiffness in my hands. Otherwise I am as healthy as anyone could wish to be. I don't remember feeling so healthy and so limber and flexible since I was a young girl."

Now in her fifties she skis regularly in winter, enjoys ocean swimming in summer, and takes long walks in the woods early in the morning before her family gets up. She also follows religiously the routines she learned at Brandal: hot and cold showers, dry brush massage, and exercises. And, naturally, she adheres faithfully to a healthful diet program which she adopted at the clinic: homemade yogurt with figs, prunes and/or raisins, plus nuts and seeds for breakfast; raw vegetable salad of all available vegetables, preferably from her own garden, for lunch; potato porridge with applesauce for dinner (see recipes in Chapter 29). In between meals, fresh unsprayed fruits plus herb teas (peppermint, camomile, or rose hips). Instead of coffee, potato and vegetable broth has become her favorite morning beverage!

Chapter 4

They Say, "There Is No Cure"

In the previous chapters you read the true stories of people who were badly crippled by arthritis. They were treated by conventional medical methods with drugs, injections, x-ray treatments, and surgery without getting better, but after changing to the biological therapies, they were completely cured. Later in this book I will show you many other cases, just as dramatic and real, taken from a long list of hundreds of actual cases which could be cited as proof that these are not isolated cases, that biological methods really work, and that arthritis sufferers indeed *can* get well!

Yet, you have read and heard on television and radio that "There is no cure for arthritis." You have been warned that anyone who speaks to the contrary must be a quack or a fraud. Americans have been brainwashed with this propaganda through various communication media for so long that they accept this statement as truth. Cleverly written and professionally acted—with the authoritative aura of white-coated actors—

these drug commercials bombard you from the magic screen day-in and day-out, in an endless repetition until you, in fatalistic resignation, giving up all hope of permanent cure, go to the nearest drugstore and buy a bottle of well-advertised painkiller, that promises you "relief."

But arthritis can be cured! Arthritis sufferers are being cured by the thousands, right now, all over the world, mostly in Europe, but also in the United States. I have seen with my own eyes how patients crippled with arthritis for years, have left their crutches and wheelchairs and walked. I have talked with and interviewed dozens of arthritics who have been cured of arthritis.

The reason why you do not hear about this from your television screen is because there is no money in selling knowledge, truth, education. You cannot pack knowledge in a bright labeled bottle, as the pill manufacturers do, and make a million dollar business out of it.

When your doctor tells you that there is no cure for arthritis he means that there is no cure for arthritis with a drug or a knife—because the pharmacological and surgical treatments are virtually the only curative methods accepted and employed by the average orthodox, allopathic medical doctor. And they are 100 per cent correct: *There is no cure for arthritis with drug or knife.*

But there definitely is a cure for arthritis with biological therapeutic methods. Thousands of arthritis sufferers throughout the world have obtained complete freedom from pain, recession of swollen joints, and disappearance of every trace of this crippling and agonizing disease. There are dozens of clinics and spas in Europe where arthritis is cured today, along with most of the other common ailments and chronic diseases. The biological methods employed by these clinics are: dietetic restrictions, fasting, herbal treatments, juice therapies, biological medicines, heat treatments, massage, manipulations, hydro-therapies, and a number of other drugless treatments. The cases cited in this book were cured by these therapies.

In the following chapters we will discuss in detail all the biological treatments which proved so successful in the reported cases, but first let us briefly analyze what arthritis is, how it develops, and why the conventional medical therapies fail to accomplish a cure.

Chapter 5

What Is Arthritis?

Arthritis is one of the oldest diseases known to man. It belongs to the "rheumatic group" of diseases which differentiate into 100 various kinds and forms of arthritic and rheumatic diseases. While the term rheumatism generally refers to the painful inflammatory conditions in the various parts of the body —like lumbago, sciatica, neuritis, etc.—the term arthritis refers specifically to inflammation of the joints.

Osteoarthritis

There are many different forms of arthritis. Perhaps the most common type is called *osteoarthritis*. It is generally considered that most people past middle age are afflicted with osteoarthritis to some extent. Osteoarthritis is usually believed to be the result of "wear and tear" on the joints during a long life. It is characterized by degenerative processes in the joints: softening and erosion of the cartilage and enlargement of the affected joints. The weight-bearing joints are usually affected first, but any joint of the body is vulnerable to osteoarthritis. One of the joints most frequently affected is the hip joint, which often becomes stiff and very painful.

Rheumatoid Arthritis

The other most common form of arthritis is *rheumatoid arthritis*. Rheumatoid arthritis is the most serious type of rheumatic affliction. It can cause severe destruction of the joint tissues which results in extensive deformations. It usually strikes younger people in early adult years, but it also can affect persons of any age. Women are afflicted with rheumatoid arthritis three times as often as men.[1] This type of arthritis starts with an inflammation of the synovial membrane, which eventually leads to deposits in the joints, bone degeneration, deformity, and subsequent invalidity if proper treatments are not instituted in time.

Gouty Arthritis

Then there is *gouty arthritis* which is usually manifested by inflammation of the joints of the large toe. This is, however, only a local symptom of a systemic, metabolic disorder of the bodily functions, usually caused by accumulation of uric acid in the tissues. Gout mainly affects men and those stricken are usually past middle age. But occasionally it may strike men and even women at an earlier age.

Mixed Arthritis

There are numerous other types of arthritis which could be classified under the common heading *mixed arthritis. Arthritis*

[1] *Arthritis*, Public Health Service Publication No. 1431, April, 1966.

deformans is a term often used to describe a certain type of arthritis. Actually, though, arthritis deformans is more a description of a condition of severe deformation from osteoarthritis, rheumatoid arthritis, and many other causes than a specific type of disease.

Ankylosing spondylitis is a vicious form of arthritis which mainly strikes down young males under the age of 20. It seldom occurs after age 30. Sacroiliac joints are the most frequent locations of spondylitis.

There are also *infectious types of arthritis* due to joint infection resulting from tuberculosis, gonorrhea, syphilis, etc.

The types of arthritis which are most topical for the purpose of this book, however, are rheumatoid arthritis and osteoarthritis. Together they are responsible for over 90 per cent of all the cases of arthritis in this country. Rheumatoid arthritis is the most painful and crippling type of them all, and it affects people of all ages, particularly those who are in their most active and productive period of life.

Symptoms

The most common symptom of arthritis is that the joints at first become painful. The pain can have many degrees of intensity and it can come and go. Sometimes it disappears for months, even years, then it returns again. At first the pain could be a feeling of numbness and stiffness. Sometimes a creaking and cracking of the joints is felt. Often the joints become swollen and inflamed. Pain can be dull but also very severe, occurring mostly at night and in the morning.

It is important to understand that these symptoms, although they may seem to be the very first signals of approaching arthritis, are not at all the first symptoms of the onset of the disease. Arthritis is not a local disease of a particular joint but a systemic disorder, a disease which affects the whole body. It could have taken years and years of abuse to bring about the

systemic disturbance in bodily functions which eventually leads
to a breakdown of the health and the functions of the joints.

How Arthritis Develops

The mechanical construction of our body allows many bones
to meet with each other in so-called joints. To avoid friction
and strain during movements, the ends of the bones are covered
with an elastic tissue called cartilage. The synovial membrane
covers the inner surfaces of the joint cavity. This membrane
secretes a fluid that lubricates the joint.

With the onset of arthritis the normal functions of the joints
are impaired. They become inflamed, enlarged, and swollen. Or
they may shrivel up and dry. The cartilages lose their elasticity
and become dry and brittle. The secretions of the synovial
membrane may diminish and with progression of the disease
cease completely. The joints thus will dry out, become congested, rough, and stiff. Also the ligaments and the muscles,
which surround the joint, become affected, inflamed, and progressively lose their tone and flexibility.

These symptoms are followed by profound and destructive
changes in the joints. Due to faulty metabolism, excessive
amounts of calcium and other minerals are deposited in the
joints. Sometimes osteoporosis, or leaching of the calcium and
other minerals from the bones, can cause severe destruction of
bones and joints.

All these changes are usually accompanied by swelling and
increasing pain during motion. Eventually the pain becomes
so unbearable that the patient will be unable to move the
affected parts of his body.

If further development is not checked and effectively treated
in time, complete destruction of the joint often will be the
ultimate result.

Many systemic disorders could be associated with the onset
of arthritis. Digestive disorders are often present in the history

of the arthritic. Constipation is often prevalent for many years before the actual arthritic symptoms begin to show up. General fatigue; physical and emotional stresses; lack of sufficient rest; nutritional deficiencies; glandular disorders, particularly in the endocrine system; unchecked infectious conditions; all could occur long before the final symptoms in the joints show up.

Therefore it is important to realize that if arthritis is to be successfully treated, the systemic nature of the disease must be recognized and the abnormal conditions and disorders of the body corrected. Unless the close relationship between the general health of the individual and his arthritis symptoms is fully recognized, all attempts to cure arthritis will be futile.

Chapter 6

What Causes Arthritis?

I have a recent newspaper clipping before me. An Associated Press correspondent reports from a medical conference, held in October, 1966 in San Francisco:

"The president of the National Arthritis Foundation, Dr. William S. Clark, says medical science will, within a relatively short time, be able to pinpoint the causes of arthritis. It could come, he said, within ten years ... Discovery of the causes of arthritis will provide the key to the cure of this disease."

That statement sums up the present stand of orthodox medicine in relation to arthritis. Medical researchers admit that they do not know what causes arthritis and, consequently, do not know how to cure it.

Biological medicine takes a much more hopeful stand on the problem of arthritis.

Although in all fairness it must be admitted that the final answers to the *exact nature and the mechanics* of the disease could not be pinpointed in detail in every case of arthritis, the empirical and practical experience of biological therapies and their positive results show that arthritis is caused by a metabolic disorder in the body. The distorted or disordered metabolism, in turn, is affected by health-destroying environmental factors, including faulty nutrition, overeating, emotional and physical stresses, sedentary life, etc.

The prevalent observation of practitioners is that the arthritic patient usually suffers from general deterioration of health in the form of sluggishness in the vital functions of his organs; incomplete digestion and assimilation of foods; impaired elimination of metabolic wastes and toxins from the system; a weakened nervous system and circulation; etc. These systemic disturbances affect the biochemical structure of the various tissues of the body. One of the pioneer practitioners of biological medicine in the United States, Dr. R. P. Watterson, M.D., calls the result of such a systemic disturbance a "biochemical suffocation." [1]

One of the most characteristic pathological changes observed in rheumatoid arthritis is the degenerative changes in collagen. [2] The changes in collagen—the connective tissues of the body, the intercellular cement—are affected by biochemical changes brought about by metabolic disorders or nutritional deficiencies. The resultant accumulation of the fibrous tissue in the joints and the accumulation of toxic wastes and mineral deposits completes the picture of a fully developed arthritis.

The reasons for the pathological degenerative changes in the tissues leading to crippling arthritis can be found in a number of man's environmental factors. Some of these are: allergic reactions; results of severe stress or injuries to the joints or related soft tissues; various kinds of infections; etc. However, by

[1] "Arthritis: Biochemical Suffocation." *Southwestern Medicine*, Vol. 42, No. 4, April, 1961.
[2] *Bircher-Benner-Handbüchlein für Rheuma-und Arthritiskranke.* Bircher-Benner Verlag, Zürich, Bad Homburg v.d.H., 1961.

far the most important causative factor in arthritis is civilized man's general deterioration of health and his diminished resistance due to faulty nutrition: overeating, malnutrition due to devitalized diet, vitamin-mineral-hormone deficiencies, etc. In addition to nutrition, other negative factors in man's environment contribute to diminished vitality and general deterioration of his health. Sedentary life with its resultant impaired circulation and anoxia; constipation; smoking and drinking; contaminated air and water; emotional and physical stresses; lack of adequate rest—all these contribute to man's bodily deterioration.

Summary

In order to understand the nature, causes, and mechanics of the development of arthritis, the following basic premises should be kept in mind:

1. Arthritis is not an unrelated, localized disease of certain joints. It is a systemic constitutional disease which always affects the whole body.

2. Arthritis is caused by metabolic disorders and systemic disturbances which effect the pathological biochemical changes in all tissues of the body, specifically in collagen.

3. These biochemical changes cause inflammatory and degenerative changes in the functions of joints and their surrounding connective tissues.

4. The underlying causes for these systemic disturbances and pathological changes are found in prolonged abuses to which the body has been subjected, such as faulty nutritional patterns, overeating, nutritional deficiencies, lack of sufficient exercise, severe emotional and physical stresses, etc. These health-destroying environmental factors eventually result in diminished vitality and lowered resistance to diseases, intestinal sluggishness, autointoxication and impaired elimination.

5. The biological treatment for arthritis is therefore aimed at the eradication and correction of all abnormal health-destroying conditions that have led to development of the disease.

6. The biological treatments are directed at normalizing all the metabolic processes; establishing biochemical stability; strengthening the functions of the vital organs; re-establishing capillary integrity; revitalizing glandular activity; and, in general, rebuilding and strengthening the general health of the patient.

7. When the causative factors are thus eliminated and the body is strengthened and revitalized by proper dietetic, physiotherapeutic, and other biological measures, then the organism's own curative powers are given a chance to take over and bring about the actual cure.

Chapter 7

Why Conventional Medical Remedies Fail

Since the average practitioner of orthodox medicine does not have a clear understanding of the basic causative principles involved in arthritis, his treatments and remedies are understandably symptomatic—that is, he is not treating the disease but the isolated symptoms of the disease. He treats an affected joint with injections, x-rays, and drugs as if it was a question of an isolated disease of the joint. He administers pain-killing drugs which will relieve pain temporarily. But, in the long run, due to their many undesirable side effects, these drugs only cause more damage and ultimately aggravate the condition instead of improving it.

As was evident from the previous chapter, arthritis is a systemic disease which affects the whole body. Therefore, the only measures that can be successful in correcting the disease, bringing it under control, and accomplishing a lasting cure, must be

33

ones directed at correcting its underlying causes. This can only be accomplished by treatments which help to overcome the systemic disturbances, normalize the metabolic processes, and help restore all normal functions of the vital organs and glands. That the conventional remedies fail to accomplish this is evident.

While drugs and injections may relieve pain and modify symptoms, they do not go to the bottom of the problem, they do not eliminate the underlying causes, nor do they correct the systemic disturbances. What is even worse, these conventional remedies, being suppressive in nature and having undesirable toxic side effects, interfere with the normal bodily processes and actually inhibit restorative and healing efforts of the body. Eventually they cause more damage than good and lead to a complete invalidism.

It must be emphatically stated that drugs do not possess curative powers. The cure is always brought about by the body itself, and the most that a wise doctor can ever do is assist the body's own healing forces. The drugs used in conventional treatment of arthritis—aspirin, cortisone, gold injections, etc.— only suppress and mask the symptoms of the disease. They do not promote the healing processes, nor do they provide any lasting benefits.

Aspirin

This "simple" and cheap remedy is used more than any other drug by millions of arthritis sufferers. The main reasons for this are: (a) aspirin is inexpensive; (b) it is easily available without prescription; (c) it is generally believed that aspirin is completely nonhabitual and harmless; and (d) it eases pain and makes the patient feel more comfortable.

Because of the above reasons aspirin is so extensively used that it is a perennial remedy and a habitual routine of virtually all arthritic patients. They use it in progressively increasing amounts and many become so dependent on aspirin that they can hardly live without the drug. Arthritics must account for a big portion of the 18 million pounds of aspirin sold in the United States yearly. Over 15 tons of aspirin is consumed every 24 hours! [1]

I wish people were better informed about how much damage this "harmless" drug can cause.

There is a general agreement among medical practitioners that aspirin is a toxic substance which has many alarming side effects.[2]

Technically known as *acetylsalicylic acid*, aspirin—and many other patented drugs which feature aspirin as a main ingredient—can cause severe poisoning and result in pathological changes in the brain, liver, and kidneys.[3]

Used over a long period of time aspirin may depress the production rate of the immune bodies of the organism and thus undermine the body's own healing powers.[4] By masking symptoms of the acute stages of arthritis, it leads the patient to a false sense of security and actually contributes to conversion of the disease to a chronic stage.

The *Journal of the American Medical Association* has reported that even small doses of aspirin can cause cardiac weakness with excessive pulse rate, edematous swelling of the mucous membranes, irregular pulse, and occasionally albuminuria (albumin in urine).[5]

Other toxic effects of aspirin are a tendency to bleed and delirium or a state of incoherency, restlessness, and confusion.

---

[1] H. Curtis Wood, Jr., M.D., *Calories, Vitamins, and Common Sense*, Belmont Books, 1962.

[2] Graham and Parker, *Quarterly Journal of Medicine*, April, 1948.

[3] "Acetylsalicylic Acid Poisoning," *Journal of the American Medical Association*, Nov. 15, 1947.

[4] Dr. Paul Dudley White, *Heart Disease*.

[5] *J.A.M.A.*, 1911.

Aspirin is also known as a vitamin antagonist. It is especially antagonistic towards vitamin C and destroys huge quantities of it in the body.[6]

This should be enough to make it clear that aspirin is far from a harmless little friend of the arthritic, as it is pictured by advertisers. Since it can cause many serious side effects and its only "good" property is in masking the symptoms, it should be evident to everyone that this remedy should not be used if the arthritis sufferer is looking for a real betterment of his condition.

The public health authorities are beginning to realize the danger of the indiscriminate use of aspirin. At a recent Surgeon General's Workshop on Prevention of Disability from Arthritis a suggestion was made "to attempt to curtail the advertising claims of salicylate derivatives so commonly heard on radio and television." [7] It was, however, agreed that such an action should come from the Federal Trade Commission's Bureau of Deceptive Practices.

Cortisone

The discovery of cortisone was hailed by medical science as one of the milestones of medical progress. We all remember, about 15 years ago, how much enthusiasm and excitement there was, both among doctors and arthritis sufferers. The world was made to believe that medical science finally had conquered this baffling disease.

It didn't take many years before it became evident that cortisone was one of those remedies which are so pertinently called "remedy worse than the disease." The "miracle" drug was found to have so many dangerous side effects that now many responsible and conscientious practitioners would not even touch it.

[6] *Nutritional Review,* 13, 46, 1955.
[7] Dr. Cornelius Traeger, M.D., *Review of Surgeon General's Workshop,* Public Health Service Publication No. 1444.

Cortisone is a hormone and is normally secreted by the adrenal glands. Now it is manufactured synthetically. Many other related hormone drugs are on the market, such as prednisone and prednisolone.

Although it is recognized that a derangement of the functions of the adrenal glands and other glands of the endocrine system contributes to the development of arthritis, the artificial use of these hormones, especially synthetically produced ones, does not mean the same as support or correction of the body's own impaired glandular functions. On the contrary, instead of rehabilitating and revitalizing the functions of the glands, these drugs only damage them further and may bring about a complete breakdown of the body's own healing powers, as far as arthritis is concerned.

Here is a partial list of side effects caused by cortisone: peptic ulcers; osteoporosis (softening of bones) with spontaneous fractures; mental disturbances; psychoses; neuropathy or the degeneration of nerves; PSC (posterior subcapsular cataracts); [8] acne; hirsutism (excessive hair growth, particularly in women); diabetes; [9] hypertension; disturbance in the metabolism and utilization of protein and fats; reactivation of tuberculosis; [10] retention of salt and water in the tissues with resultant strain on heart and kidneys; [11] probable reduction of resistance to carcinogenesis (susceptibility to cancer); [12] etc.

This list should be enough to discourage anybody from using this dangerous drug. It can damage the liver, the kidneys, the blood, the bones, the nerves, as well as other vital organs of the body.

[8] *Journal of A.M.A.*, Sept. 10, 1966. Editorial.
[9] "A New Drug is Born," *Journal of A.M.A.*, Sept. 24, 1960.
[10] Max Warmbrand, N.D., D.O., *Arthritis Sufferers Can Get Well*, Hovarth Publications, Inc.
[11] *U.S. News and World Report*, June 3, 1955. From the statement by Dr. Floyd S. Daft, Director of the National Institute of Arthritis.
[12] R. P. Watterson, M.D., "Arthritis, Biochemical Suffocation," *Southwestern Medicine*, Vol. 42, No. 4, April, 1961.

Worst of all, cortisone therapy causes adrenal atrophy and undermines and disturbs the entire biochemical stability of the arthritic patient.[13] Corticosteroid therapy has a damaging effect on the joints [12] and can cause deterioration of the tissues of the joints.[13] Once cortisone is taken or injected over any appreciable length of time, it will cause such a breakdown of the organs and the functions of the body that often it will be impossible to bring the patient back to a state of health again. The Swedish doctors, Karl-Otto Aly, M.D., Lars-Erik Essén, M.D., and Jern Hamberg, M.D.—the pioneers of biological medicine in Sweden, whom I spoke with in regard to cortisone therapy—all unanimously stated that by far the worst adverse effect of cortisone therapy, even worse than its toxic side effects, is its damaging and undermining effect on the body's own healing activity. It is very difficult, often impossible, to successfully employ biological treatments and restore a patient to complete health if he has used cortisone for any extended period of time.

Cortisone is a diabolical drug. It suppresses symptoms of arthritis so well that the patient believes it has made him well— suddenly he can walk, run, dance. But this is only for a moment. When the effect of cortisone wears off, the patient feels worse than ever. So he becomes addicted to it, and the withdrawal symptoms grow more painful the longer he uses it. Discontinuance of cortisone therapy is, therefore, accompanied by a great deal of suffering.

It is evident from the above why cortisone failed to fulfill its early promise and why now it can be counted out as an effective arthritis remedy.

Gold Injections

Gold therapy has been greatly popularized and acclaimed as one of the most effective remedies for arthritis. Exactly how

[13] *Journal of A.M.A.*, August 27, 1960.

the injected gold salts work in the body is not known. Nor is it known how the body reacts to them. Since gold therapy produces some relief of the symptoms it is believed that it acts as a stimulant on the vital processes of the body.

Gold injections, however, are known to be highly toxic and may produce many diseases and complications. Liver and kidneys can be seriously damaged, which may even cause death.[14] Various skin diseases are a common result of gold injections. Stomach disorders, deafness, anemia, hemorrhages under the skin, neuritis, headache, eye impairments, ulcerations of the mouth and gums [15]—these are just a few of the most serious diseases caused by gold therapy. In fact the toxic nature of gold salts and the dangers of gold treatments are so well recognized by physicians that it is usually recommended only in cases where other forms of treatment have completely failed.

As in the case of aspirin and cortisone, gold injections do not go to the bottom of the problem; they do not eliminate or alleviate the basic causative factors of the disease. Considering the grave risks involved in its use, gold therapy should have been abandoned long ago as a remedy for arthritis.

New drugs are constantly developed by pharmaceutical companies searching for a miracle drug which will cure arthritis. Indomethacin is one drug which is considered by the National Institute of Arthritis and Metabolic Diseases as the most promising at the present time. Other recently developed drugs are phenylbutazone and unpronounceable triethylene-thiophosphoramide. All are potent pain-killers with equally potent side effects.

As I mentioned before, all these conventional treatments and remedies have failed to bring about a real, permanent bet-

[14] Dr. William B. Rawls, "An Evaluation of the Present-Day Therapy in Rheumatoid Arthritis," *New York Medicine*, August 5, 1947.
[15] Max Warmbrand, N.D., D.O., *The Encyclopedia of Natural Health*, Groton Press, Inc.

terment and cure for arthritis. The reason for this is obvious: Orthodox medicine, by its own admission, does not know the cause of arthritis. Since they don't know what causes arthritis, it would then be logical to expect that they don't know what to do or how to go about finding a cure.

Chapter 8

The Program of Biological
Treatments

In Chapter 6 I have shown that biological medicine sees arthritis as a systemic disease caused by metabolic disorder and chemical imbalance in the organs, glands, and tissues of the body. The inflammatory and the degenerative changes in the functions of the joints and the surrounding tissues are brought about by the biochemical disturbance, hormonal imbalance, and weakened functions of the vital organs, effected by the prolonged physical and emotional abuses and stresses to which the body has been subjected.

The biological therapies, therefore, are directed at: (1) eradication and correction of the abnormal and health-destroying conditions which have led to the development of the disease; (2) assisting the body's own healing forces in normalizing all the metabolic processes, cleansing the body of the accumulated toxins and wastes, strengthening the functions of all the vital organs, revitalizing the glandular activity, establishing a chemical balance in the tissues—or, in sum total, *rebuilding and strengthening the general health of the patient.*

Withdrawal of Drugs

Because conventional drugs used in medical treatment of arthritis are, as a rule, only aimed at masking and suppressing the symptoms, they naturally have no place in a program of biological treatments. Pain is an important symptom, a signal, which is initiated by the body's own defensive mechanism to attract necessary help and assistance for its healing activity. To suppress and mask pain, without finding out why it is there and trying to eliminate the underlying causes of it, is contrary to the philosophy of biological medicine. It is of vital importance to realize that the various symptoms of disease, such as pain, swelling, stiffness, fever, tiredness, loss of appetite, etc. are not negative phenomena which have to be eliminated and suppressed, but they are positive, constructive symptoms initiated by the body's own healing mechanism in its effort to restore health. When this is clearly understood, then the wise doctor will not waste his own and his patient's time masking the symptoms and providing temporary relief. He will adopt a positive attitude which will aim at eliminating and correcting the underlying causative factors of arthritis and supporting the body's own recuperative powers.

Even such a drug as cortisone, although it will temporarily activate and stabilize the chemical balance of the tissues, will never correct the initial disturbance and will eventually cause more damage by undermining and impairing the body's own corrective measures. Therefore, cortisone, like any other toxic drug, should be used only in a situation of extreme emergency.

Consequently, the first rule of a biological program is complete withdrawal of all drugs. In the great majority of cases this presents no problems. Naturally, withdrawal of pain-killing drugs will cause a certain amount of discomfort for the first few days, but on a new biological program the patient soon will be pain-free, even without pain-killing drugs.

The consensus of opinion of doctors who use biological methods in their practice is that the prospects of achieving a betterment and cure of arthritis with the help of biological treatments is in inverse relationship to the extent and intensity of the drug treatment the patient received previously.[1,2] Prolonged use of drugs will eventually suppress and break down the body's own defense and healing mechanisms causing severe chemical and hormonal imbalance. The disease will then be pushed further and further towards the condition where it will be completely incurable.[1]

Therefore, in order to obtain lasting results the withdrawal of all drugs is imperative.

Diet

Because the underlying causes of arthritis are to be found in the degenerative changes brought about by faulty living habits and specifically by nutritional abuses, it stands to reason to expect that a program of biological treatments is dominated by dietetic measures.

It is a general observation that the diet of arthritic patients has been deficient in vital nutritive elements for prolonged periods and loaded with overcooked, canned, frozen, devitalized, and overrefined foods. In addition, the great amount of empty calories from white sugar and white flour and all the foodless monstrosities made from them makes such a diet even

[1] *Vidi Nova*, No. 1, 1964-1965, page 22: *"The more extensive* the chemical treatment—*the less* possibility for recovery."
[2] "Arthritis: Biochemical Suffocation," *Southwestern Medicine*, Vol. 42, No 4, April, 1961.

more unhealthy. This sort of nutritional abuse, combined with other health-destroying factors in the form of overeating, use of alcohol, smoking, coffee, lack of exercise, etc., has caused a general breakdown of their health and triggered the development of degenerative processes in their joints.

In order to reverse the process, rebuild the general health of the patient, initiate a betterment in his condition, and induce a subsequent cure, a radical overhaul of his dietary habits is of prime importance. The diet must be as easy as possible for the digestive system to handle and, at the same time, provide all the nutrients required for the repair and building of a healthy body.

The diet during the first two to four weeks consists mainly of raw, uncooked fruits and vegetables (Frischkost). Some of the clinics which I visited use certain amounts of cooked foods in addition to Frischkost. Most Swedish biological clinics use boiled potatoes and vegetable soups in addition to raw foods. They all use raw milk in the form of homemade soured milk. The Bircher-Benner Clinic in Switzerland, one of the most advanced and best-known biological clinics in the world, excludes all cooked foods during the first phase of the treatment—as well as all foods of animal origin: meat, fish, eggs, milk, butter, and cheese. Bread and cooked cereals are eliminated as well during the first two to four weeks. Raw nuts, seeds, and sprouted grains are included in the raw food diet.

Uncooked foods will supply not only all the necessary vitamins and minerals, but also all the enzymes and easily digestible natural starches and proteins needed for healthy functioning of the body. Another advantage of such a diet is that it will cause a minimum of waste retention and sluggishness in the digestive organs and will help the body in its cleansing and detoxicating process. It is a purifying and cleansing diet. (See next chapter for a detailed description of optimum nutrition for optimum health.)

Therapeutic Fasting

The rudimentary biological measure considered fundamental by most clinics successfully applying biological principles in the treatment of arthritis is fasting.

Although fasting is one of the oldest therapeutic methods known to man and has been a dependable curative measure throughout medical history, the present drug-oriented, orthodox medical doctor has little understanding, and even less appreciation, of its remarkable benefits.

Biologically oriented doctors, however, consider fasting to be singularly the most important curative measure in treatment of arthritis. Some of them disagree as to the length of fasting, but all of them, without exception, use fasts in their program of treatments.

Dr. Otto Buchinger, Jr., M.D., of Klinik Dr. Buchinger, Forstweb 39, 3280, Bad Pyrmont, Germany, is perhaps the world's foremost authority on fasting. He has experience with over 50,000 fasts which he and his father, Dr. Otto Buchinger, Sr., directed and supervised at their clinics. At present his sanatorium accepts 85 patients ranging from afflictions of arthritis to high blood pressure; cancer; liver, kidney, and bladder diseases; and practically any other kind of known disease. Of these, 90 percent are treated by fasts, ranging from one week to 60 days.

Similarly, all Swedish clinics use fasts in their programs. Dr. Lars-Erik Essén, M.D. of the Vita Nova Clinic in Mölle, Sweden, is one who takes exception to the long fasting for arthritis. He recommends repeated short fasts—three to five days at a time—followed by a special cleansing diet. The other Swedish clinics—Brandals, Björkagården, Dr. Jern Hamberg's Alfta Clinic, Kiholms, and others—use fasts of one to six weeks' duration.

How the Fast Works

Therapeutic fasting is a total abstinence from food. The purpose of fast is to promote healing and restore health.

Therapeutic values of fasting are well documented by a large number of scientific investigations, studies, research, and practical observation. Doctors who employ fasting testify that it indeed "works." As Dr. Adolph Mayer asserted, "Fasting is the most efficient means of correcting any disease." [3]

But how can mere abstinence from food accomplish such remarkable healing results?

The therapeutic value of fasting is based on the following physiological facts:

1. Autolysis is a known metabolic phenomenon of self-digestion or disintegration of the body's own tissues.

2. Therapeutic fasting induces the development of autolysis and directs its physiological effect for constructive healing purposes.

To clarify: when disease takes hold of the body it is usually because of the weakened defensive mechanism and impaired normal functions of the vital organs. Due to continuous neglect in feeding the body properly and failure to observe the other rules of health, the glandular activity and metabolic rate slows down and the eliminative organs lose their efficiency. Many of the toxins and metabolic wastes remain in the body and are deposited in the tissues, causing autointoxication. In rheumatic diseases these wastes, such as uric acid crystals and mineral compounds, are deposited in the joints and soft tissues. In the case of high blood pressure, these metabolic wastes are deposited in arteries and small blood capillaries, constricting them and hindering the normal flow of blood. In self-defense the

[3] Arnold De Vries, *Therapeutic Fasting,* Chandler Book Co., Los Angeles, 1963.

heart increases arterial and capillary pressure to push blood through the plugged vessels.

Now, we must recognize the fact that the body's own healing powers are constantly trying to correct any and all defects, disturbances, and damages if given the slightest chance. Such a chance and opportunity for self-regeneration and healing is made possible during the fast.

First, during prolonged fast (after the first three days) the body will burn and digest its own tissues by the process of autolysis, or self-digestion. In its wisdom—and here lies the secret of the extraordinary effectiveness of fasting as curative therapy!— the body will only decompose and burn those substances and tissues which are diseased, damaged, or of lesser importance to the body economy, such as all morbid accumulations, tumors, abscesses, damaged tissues, fat deposits, etc. These are consumed and utilized first. The essential tissues of vital organs are spared.

Second, the eliminating and cleansing capacity of the eliminative organs—lungs, liver, kidneys, and skin—is increased during fasting, and masses of accumulated metabolic wastes and toxins are quickly expelled. This is evident in the following typical symptoms of fasting: offensive breath, dark urine (concentration of toxins in urine ten times higher than normal— Professor E. G. Schonk),[4] continuous and generous discharge of feces, skin eruptions, perspiration, catarrhal elimination, etc.

Third, a fast affords a physiological rest to the digestive and protective organs of the body. After fasting, the digestion and utilization of food is greatly improved, which makes the assimilation of all the important nutrients more effective.

Fourth, a fast exerts a normalizing and stabilizing effect on all the physiological, nervous, and mental functions. The nerv-

[4] Arnold De Vries, *Therapeutic Fasting,* Chandler Book Co., Los Angeles, 1963.

ous system is regenerated; mental powers improved; glandular chemistry and secretions are normalized.

It is easy to see, then, why fasting is such an effective therapeutic measure in treatment of a great variety of diseases, including arthritis.

Later in the book I will describe in detail how fasting is carried out in Swedish clinics (Chapter 11) and how it can be done in your own home (Chapter 17).

Fresh Juices

Although the classic form of fasting is the so-called pure water fast (abstinence from all foods and drinks with the exception of pure water), all the practitioners I interviewed in European clinics, including the champion of therapeutic fasting in modern times, Dr. Otto Buchinger, Jr., use fresh juices, vegetable broths, and herb teas during fasting.

Biologically oriented doctors feel that freshly pressed vegetable and fruit juices, given to the patient during fast, will speed his recovery. This is attributed to the fact that raw vegetable and fruit juices, as well as freshly made vegetable broth, are rich in vitamins, minerals, enzymes, and trace elements, which help to normalize the bodily processes and speed up recovery. At the same time, they are very easily assimilated directly into the bloodstream without putting a strain on the digestive organs.

Juices most frequently used in Sweden are: carrot juice, apple juice, black currant juice, and tomato juice.

Vegetable Broth

Vegetable broth is made by boiling all kinds of available vegetables, but predominantly potatoes, carrots, and celery, chopped to about half-inch pieces, for 30 minutes in a pot of water. (Use only stainless steel, glass, or earthenware utensils.)

Then it is strained and the vegetables are thrown away. The remaining liquid is a highly alkaline, mineral-packed broth, which is considered to be of extraordinary importance in biological arthritis therapy. It combats acidosis or a tendency toward a high acidity in the bloodstream and tissues. It helps to normalize the mineral balance in the tissues, which, according to Dr. Lars-Erik Essén, is of utmost importance for the effectiveness of the fast.

Both vegetable broth and fresh vegetable and fruit juices are concentrated nutrition. Perhaps, it would be more appropriate to call such therapy a liquid diet, rather than a fast.

Herb Teas

All biological clinics use various herb teas, both during fasting and while on a diet.

The medicinal value of herbs is well known. Herb medicines are the oldest remedy known to man.

The herb teas used in Swedish clinics are usually made from native herbs: rose hips (very rich in vitamin C), peppermint, milfoil, etc. Swedish health food stores are well stocked with dozens of herb teas, many of them combinations of different herbs mixed for specific diseases.

Enema

Fasting is always accompanied by enemas, or colonic baths, taken two or three times a day. Most clinics administer an enema twice a day; some, like Björkagården and Vita Nova, three times a day, two or three small enemas at a time. An enema is generally considered to be an extremely important measure for keeping the large intestine clean from wastes and speeding evacuation of toxic matter from the system through the bowels.

Intermediate Diet

After the fast is broken, the patient is put on a special diet. This consists of an abundance of raw vegetables and fruits, vegetable and fruit juices, some cooked dishes, such as boiled potatoes, vegetable soups, beans, homemade soured milk (from raw unpasteurized milk), whey cheese, and salt-free cottage cheese.

Colonic Irrigation

In addition to an enema the patients who have a record of chronic constipation prior to coming to the clinic (a common affliction of many arthritics) are given a colonic irrigation once or twice during the first week. This is a treatment which employs a specially constructed appliance to thoroughly wash the large intestine and colonic tract.

Hot and Cold Shower

One of the treatments which many practitioners, particularly at the Brandals Clinic, attach a great importance to, is an alternating hot and cold shower. It is administered in the morning.

The procedure is as follows: First, a warm shower for about ten to 15 minutes to get the body really warmed up. This is followed by a cold shower for approximately one to three minutes. Water should be as cold as the patient can stand. After that the patient receives a vigorous dry brushing with a stiff brush and is rubbed with a coarse towel until he is completely warmed up.

The importance of the alternating hot and cold shower lies in the fact that it stimulates the adrenal and other endocrine glands and reactivates their functions. Alma Nissen calls such a shower "a cortisone injection—but without cortisone's undesirable side effects!"

Sufficient Rest

All biological clinics stress the importance of sufficient rest for patients with arthritis. After lunch, 1:00 P.M. to 3:00 P.M., there is an obligatory quiet hour, when all patients take a long afternoon nap.

Exercise

Various therapeutic exercises are a standard routine in the biological clinic. Exercises are adapted to the condition of the patient. Walks in the woods are encouraged—all the Swedish clinics which I visited are surrounded by beautiful woods that afford invigorating walks in the fresh air. In addition, special relaxation gymnastics are given in some clinics.

Baths

Therapeutic baths are an important part of the biological program. In addition to alternating hot and cold showers, mentioned before, the following baths are employed: whirlpool massage, sitz bath, Kuhne-bath, steam bath, sauna, Güsseshower, warm sand bath (Bircher-Benner), etc.

Massage

Dry brush massage is an important therapeutic measure. It stimulates the circulation; brings the blood to the skin; keeps skin clean from dead cells and impurities; and opens the pores. The skin is your biggest eliminative organ and it is of vital importance that it functions as such efficiently.

In addition, conventional massage—so-called Swedish massage—is frequently used to help the affected joints to regain their lost elasticity and movements.

Many Other Forms

Many other forms of biological treatments are used in addition to the "standards" outlined above. Every clinic has its own specialties. Björkagården stresses vacuum massage and modern cupping as being of extraordinary importance. Vita Nova uses nontoxic biological medicines in the form of subcutaneous injections. Various forms of heat treatments are used in almost all clinics: high-frequency, pulsed, short-wave therapy; infrared heat lamps; cold and hot packs; mud packs (Heilerde); etc.

Positive Attitude

The importance of proper attitude on the part of patients is emphasized in all clinics. After years of pain and suffering, persons afflicted with arthritis are often irritable, tense, bitter, and resentful. These negative emotions can do much to make efforts to regain health difficult, even impossible.

Therefore, fostering a positive, trustful attitude in the patient and insuring his thorough understanding of the various biological treatments and expected reactions is a very important part of the total program in every biological clinic. Several evenings every week special lectures are presented to acquaint new patients with the intricate metabolic processes of the body and the functions of various organs. The causative factors leading to the development of the disease are explained. The mechanics and effects of biological treatments, as well as the whole philosophy of biological medicine, is made clear and comprehensive. The fact that there are no shortcuts to the cure of arthritis is emphasized. A biological program of treatments is not easy. There are no specific miracle treatments, no specific diets which can cure arthritis. Arthritis can be cured only by the efforts of the body's own healing powers. With the assistance of the wide arsenal of biological treatments and with the full and cheerful cooperation of the patient it can be done. It is done every day. But in order to achieve lasting and effective results, full cooperation and a positive effort on the part of the patient is imperative.

The patient must understand that the cure is possible only if he is willing to discard completely his former mode of living and accept a new way of life. He must have the willingness and determination to follow the new biological programs and have a trustful and cooperative attitude. The negative attitude will lock up the healing forces of the body, whereas a positive attitude will unlock them and spur them into full action.

It requires a certain amount of intelligence, understanding, and patience, in addition to a sense of determination and self-discipline, to undertake a biological program of treatments and not give up before noticeable results are observed. It often takes time to induce a betterment.

The doctor of a biological clinic lives up to the letter of his true call: to be a *teacher* (*doctor* means *teacher* in Latin). He teaches his patients a new way of life. He inspires them to a better, more healthful mode of living. The patient must learn that arthritis is not an isolated disease but is a result of general health deterioration. He must clearly see that in order to correct his disease, the whole body must be regenerated and rebuilt. No drug can possibly accomplish this. Only biological methods can and do regenerate and rebuild the whole system and, thus, help the body's own healing forces to correct arthritis and restore health.

Biological Methods Scientifically Proven

By now it must be evident to the average reader that the biological approach to arthritis is quite different from conventional practices. As with every new concept and new approach, it takes an unprejudiced and objective attitude on the part of practitioners to be able to grasp and accept the new discoveries. It is natural to be doubtful and even skeptical of something which is contrary to common practice and the accepted line of thought. Moreover, the new biological approach seems to be so down-to-earth simple that for a technologically minded and pseudoscientifically trained, twentieth century space-oriented man it may seem too simple to be true. However, hundreds of medical doctors in Europe have given this down-to-earth, commonsense, nature-cure approach a fair trial. They were soon convinced of its extraordinary merits. Its effectiveness is proven by actual result-producing application on thousands upon thousands of successfully treated patients.

The value of biological treatments was scientifically tested by the Royal Free Hospital in London, England, in 1949. The experiments were made through the initiative of one of the hospital doctors who had seen a successfully treated case of arthritis. The methods used were those employed at the famous Bircher-Benner Clinic in Switzerland.

Twelve patients with arthritis, all more or less hopeless cases given up by doctors as not responsive to conventional treatments, were selected to participate in the tests, which were carried out under careful scientific control. The experiment was documented on films taken during the entire duration of the tests, and a detailed report was given in a medical journal.[5]

The results of the experiment were very convincing. Patients who were considered hopeless cases had remarkably improved and regained the use of their deformed and formerly immobile joints.

One 55-year-old woman was so badly crippled that she could hardly move any part of her body and was permanently bedridden. After less than one year on the biological program, she

[5] *Proceedings of the Royal Society of Medicine*, Vol. XXX.

left the hospital walking without help and without crutches. This case was controlled ten years later (1959) and the patient, now at the age of 65, was found in good health, able to do hard physical labor, such as digging in her garden two or three hours without rest.

It is unfortunate, indeed, that it takes such a long time before new discoveries and original ideas become universally accepted and officially endorsed. Millions of sick people suffer because of unwillingness on the part of conservative practitioners to accept and use new, unconventional methods of treatment. It is my sincere hope that this book will spread the knowledge and speed the recognition of biological medicine, both among the members of the healing professions as well as the lay public, and help to free millions of arthritis sufferers from their hopelessness and agonizing existence.

Chapter 9

The Vital Role of Nutrition

As you have learned from previous chapters, faulty nutrition is singularly the most important causative factor in the development of arthritis. An unbalanced diet of devitalized, over-processed, overcooked, and overrefined denatured foods combined with toxic and foodless items such as tobacco, alcohol, coffee, sugar, salt, irritating spices, chocolate, soft drinks, sweets, pastries, pies, etc., together with other negative environmental factors, brings about a general deterioration of health, biochemical imbalance, and systemic disturbances. These deleterious factors eventually lead to a total metabolic disorder and consequent pathological changes in the joints and tissues of the body.

Therefore, tne first step in an effective program of treatment for arthritis must be a complete change of nutritional patterns. Arthritis can be conquered only by rebuilding and restoring the general health of the patient. The functions of his vital organs must be strengthened; the glandular activity stimulated; the eliminative processes activated; and the digestion and assimilation improved. All this can be done only from within with vital nutritive elements needed for the repair and rebuilding processes within the body.

It should not be too difficult to see that proper nutrition is the most important factor in restoring health. The question is: What is proper nutrition?

You may say, "I have been health conscious for a long time. I eat plenty of meat and eggs and drink lots of milk for my protein. I eat cereal for breakfast and one or two vegetables with my meat each day. And I take a one-a-day vitamin tablet each day, too." This description of a "health" diet would about sum up the average American concept of proper nutrition: lots of animal protein; devitalized, foodless cereals; canned vegetables and instant mashed potatoes; white bread; sugared desserts out of the can ... It is a miracle that not more than 8 to 10 per cent of the American people develop arthritis on such a monstrous diet! And yet, most Americans actually believe that they are the best fed nation in the world. Perhaps they are the best fed quantitatively speaking, but certainly not the best nourished!

There is much disagreement and confusion, even among the prominent nutritionists, as to what constitutes a wholesome diet. Many theories exist and too many popular or pseudo-scientific books are written to further confuse the issues. No wonder the average man is puzzled and confused.

On the basis of existing empirical and scientific evidence, the wholesome food program of vital nutrition with the greatest potential for optimum health and prevention of disease should comply with the following seven basic rules:

1. Natural Foods

The first and most important principle of optimum nutrition is that you should eat natural foods.

Natural foods are foods grown under natural conditions in man's natural environment, consumed in their natural state. It would be unnatural for an Eskimo to live on a raw vegetarian diet, just as it is unnatural for inhabitants of tropical or sub-tropical regions to eat meat.

Dr. Weston A. Price made an extensive study of health and diet habits of practically every race of people in the world and came to the conclusion that the condition of their health is in direct relation to the "naturalness" of the foods they eat.[1] Wherever he found strong, healthy people without diseases and without tooth decay, he learned that their diets were made up of natural, fresh, pure, and unprocessed foods, available in their immediate environment. Conversely, where he found people subject to dental decay and various diseases common to civilized man, he invariably discovered that they ate denatured, cooked, processed foods and that white sugar, white bread, canned foods, etc. had found their way to them from more "civilized" countries.

In the United States, we have departed so far from the natural way of life that for many it is difficult to comprehend what is meant by natural foods.

Let's clarify this with an example. Eggs laid by hens which have access to the outdoors, green grass, seeds, insects, and worms are *natural*, fertile eggs full of nutritive value. But eggs produced in an egg factory, by hens who never see a rooster, nor sunlight, and eat only synthetic mash, are not natural. Not only is the chemical composition of such an egg altered and unbalanced, but also its nutritional value is far below that of a natural egg.

Natural fruits and vegetables should grow in healthy, fertile soils, without chemical fertilizers or sprays. Equally, animal food

[1] Weston A. Price, D.D.S., *Nutrition and Physical Degeneration*, Lee Foundation for Nutritional Research, 2023 W. Wisconsin Ave., Milwaukee, Wisconsin

—milk, cheese, or meat—should come from healthy animals which are fed organically grown fodder and are not artificially raised with the help of hormones, antibiotics, and poisonous chemicals.

Natural foods contain more vitamins, more proteins, more minerals and other nutrients, particularly the vital enzymes, than denatured foods.

The human body is a living organism, a part of the complex organic universe subject to the unchangeable laws of nature. The human body must have living, organic food elements in their unaltered natural state in order to survive and live in good health. Synthetic, altered, poisoned, processed, and devitalized foods will not sustain health, but will bring about a degeneration of normal bodily functions and disease.

2. Whole Foods

The second rule of vital nutrition is that your foods should be whole, complete, unrefined, and unadulterated. Whole wheat, brown rice, orange, sugar cane, and potatoes are whole foods. White bread, polished rice, orange juice, white sugar, and instant potatoes are not whole foods. They are refined, concentrated, or are fragments of the foods from which important vital nutritive factors have been removed.

Whole foods are simply foods which still contain all the nutrients which nature has put in them—all the vitamins, minerals, proteins, carbohydrates, enzymes, etc. But 80 per cent of the foods consumed by the average American today have been tampered with in one way or another, and most of the nutrients have either been taken out of them or destroyed. White bread, white sugar, breakfast cereals, and processed oils are typical examples of such devitalized nutritionless foods.

Whole foods contain not only complete nutrition but also all the enzymes and other factors necessary for proper digestion and good assimilation of these particular foods. When certain parts are removed, the digestion and assimilation can be incomplete and nutritional deficiences may result.

Only whole foods can supply optimum nutrition for optimum health.

3. Living Foods

The third rule of vital nutrition is that all foods should be eaten as fresh as possible. Fruits and vegetables should be eaten raw, not cooked, canned, or frozen. If cooking is necessary they should be cooked as little as possible, preferably steamed or cooked with little or no water. All broth, of course, should be used also.

Raw foods contain enzymes which are essential for the proper digestion and assimilation of food. Cooking destroys all the enzymes, 100 per cent. In addition, cooking destroys many of the vitamins. Vitamins B and C are particularly vulnerable to the effects of heat. Minerals are depleted by cooking and are usually thrown away with the cooking water.

Freezing, canning, drying, salting, preserving, and prolonged storage are all more or less destructive to the nutritive quality of the food.

Contrary to popular notion, foods in their raw state are more easily digestible than in the cooked state. This is particularly true with fruits and most vegetables.

Furthermore, raw foods act as a cleansing agent of the digestive and eliminative systems and are the best preventive measures against constipation.

Dr. Robert Bell hit the nail on the head when he said, "Man is the only creature upon this earth who spoils his food before he eats it." Cooked food is dead food. Only living foods can build healthy bodies.

According to famous nutritionist Dr. Royal Lee, D.D.S., arthritis in animals could be experimentally caused by feeding them cooked foods exclusively.

4. Poison-Free Foods

The fourth rule of vital nutrition is that your food should be as poison-free as possible. This is easier said than done, however, in this poisoned world of ours. And if you feel that "poisoned world" sounds rather alarmist, I will add that it is almost impossible these days in the United States and West-European countries to obtain foodstuffs that are free from poisonous residues or additives. Fruits and vegetables contain residues of various poisonous insecticides, waxes, bleaches, and artificial colorings. Fresh meats contain residues of hormones used to speed up animal growth and antibiotics to prolong meat's shelf life. Processed meats, bread, cereals, canned and processed foods are loaded with some of the nearly 1,000 different chemicals now used by the food processing industry in this country—and many of them have never been tested for their possible toxicity! Much recent research shows that the toxic effect of chemicals is multiplied by the effect of other chemical agents consumed simultaneously.

There is a growing movement in the United States to produce poison-free, organically grown foods. They are often available in health food stores. Every effort should be made to obtain such foods. Poisons in foods are, perhaps, the greatest menace to American health today.

5. Balanced Diet

The worn-out cliché, "the balanced diet," has been so misused and abused that it no longer has much meaning. The term *optimum diet* would better signify a diet so well planned and chosen as to assure optimum health.

What is a balanced diet? Is it a diet made up of "four basic foods" as you were taught in grade school? Or is it the "seven basics" as it is sometimes advised? Whichever it is, meat has always been considered the most basic food. We have all been brainwashed for years with the pseudoscientific slogan *"high protein—low carbohydrate."* We believe that we should eat as much protein as possible. We are living in an era of the high-protein cult!

When I recently met Dr. Karl-Otto Aly, M.D., the prominent Swedish doctor, upon his return from an extensive lecture tour in the United States and asked him, "What is singularly the most memorable impression of your trip?" he had an immediate answer:

"The American high-protein craze! Not only the general public, but even so-called health enthusiasts are so thoroughly brainwashed on the question of protein in their diet, that, to my mind, this point alone may be held responsible to a great degree for the deplorable state of health of the American people."

In Chapter 22 I will answer in more detail the question: Should arthritis sufferers adhere to a high-protein diet? Also, I will attempt to solve the mystery of the American high-protein myth. In the meantime, let me categorically state that the latest scientific findings, as well as practical empirical experience, points out the undisputable fact that the optimum diet for optimum health and vitality is a diet *low in animal protein* and *rich in natural carbohydrates and protein foods from vegetable sources.* Such a diet would include raw fruits and vegetables, nuts and seeds, whole grains, milk and milk products; these nutritious foods should be fortified with wheat germ, brewer's yeast, cold-pressed vegetable oils, honey, and powdered skim milk. The above foods constitute a well-balanced diet which will supply you not only with essential vitamins, minerals, carbohydrates, trace elements, and enzymes, but with all the necessary complete proteins as well.

6. Undereating

The latest scientific research shows that the single most important health and longevity factor is a scanty diet or underfeeding. Statistics collected from the several thousands of centenarians in Russia show that one common characteristic of all people who lived 100 years or longer is that throughout their lives they were all moderate eaters. Extensive animal studies reveal that moderate underfeeding increases longevity and decreases incidence of degenerative diseases.[2] The eminent scientist, Dr. C. M. McCays of Cornell University, has shown by his research that overeating is the major cause of premature aging in civilized countries. To prolong life and assure good health he recommends a scanty diet of nutritionally superior natural foods.

As Benjamin Franklin said, "A full belly is the mother of all evil." Obesity is, perhaps, the biggest American health problem and a contributing cause in the contraction of many diseases, including arthritis. As Thomas Edison suggested, "People gorge themselves with rich foods, use their time, ruin their digestion, and poison themselves . . ."

Food eaten in excess of the actual bodily need acts in the system as a poison; interferes with digestion; causes internal sluggishness, gas, incomplete assimilation, and other metabolic disturbances. It causes fermentation and putrefaction and actually poisons your system.

Leave your table when the food tastes its best. Several smaller meals or snacks are better than a few huge meals. Train yourself to systematically undereat and you will give yourself the best—and the cheapest—health insurance possible.

7. Correct Eating Habits

And lastly, not only *what* you eat, but *how* you eat is extremely important. After all, we are not what we eat, but what we assimilate. And assimilation of nutrients from the foods you eat is to a large degree dependent on proper eating habits.

Many of us eat too fast, gulp our food down without chewing it properly—not to mention the fact that we often eat when we

[2] *Canadian Medical Association Journal*, Oct. 23, 1965.

are not really hungry, merely because it is dinner time. Also, we eat when we are tense and irritated or when our thoughts are far away from food. Or, we eat certain foods because we think they are good for us, without really enjoying them.

No, all foods should be eaten slowly and chewed very thoroughly. Never eat in a hurry. It is far better to skip a meal than to eat it in a hurry. Slow eating and good mastication will increase the assimilation of nutrients in the intestinal tract and make you feel satisfied with a smaller quantity of food. Well-chewed and generously salivated food is practically half-digested in the mouth. Saliva contains enzymes and other digestive agents.

And, finally, food should be eaten in a relaxed atmosphere and enjoyed. My old friend and teacher, Dr. Ragnar Berg, one of the world's most renowned nutritionists, used to say, "Eating should be a pleasure." Please, don't misconstrue his statement to mean that you should eat *for* pleasure! Eat to live—don't live to eat! The biological fact is that only foods eaten with a genuine pleasure will do you any good. A peaceful, unhurried, pleasurable, and happy atmosphere around the table will pay good dividends in improved digestion and assimilation of food and in better health.

The Menu

In accordance with the above seven rules of vital nutrition, your menu for a well-balanced, wholesome diet for optimum health and prevention of disease should look approximately like this:

UPON ARISING: Glass of water, plain, or with freshly squeezed lemon juice.

OR: Big cup of warm herb tea. Choice of rose hips, peppermint, camomile, maté, or any other herb tea.*

* See Chapter 29 for recipe.

OR: Glass of freshly made fruit juice: orange, apple, pineapple, etc. No canned or frozen juices. Juice should be freshly made on your own juicer from the available fresh fruits. Juice should be diluted with water, half and half. (Do not confuse a juicer with a blender. Juicers cost approximately $60 and make a pulp-free juice.)

BREAKFAST: Fresh fruit: apple, orange, banana, grapes, grapefruit, or other fruits.
Cup of yogurt or homemade soured milk * (made from raw, unpasteurized milk) with tablespoon of raw wheat germ, tablespoon of sunflower meal, and/or tablespoon of flaxseed meal sprinkled over.

OR: Bowl of rolled oats, uncooked, with 4-6 soaked prunes (or 2-3 figs) and handful of unsulfured raisins.
Glass of unpasteurized milk.

OR: Bowl of Bircher-Benner Müesli.*

OR: Bowl of cooked oatmeal, or other whole grain cereal with soaked prunes and unsulfured raisins.
Glass of milk.

OR: Fresh fruit after season.
Glass of nut-milk or banana shake.*

LUNCH: Big bowl of fresh, green vegetable salad.*
2 or 3 middle-sized potatoes or 1 big sweet potato, boiled or baked in jackets.
1-2 slices of whole wheat bread or sour

* See Chapter 29 for recipe.

bread * with butter and mild natural cheese.

Glass of yogurt or homemade soured milk.

OR: Big bowl of fresh Fruit Salad à la Airola.*

OR: Bowl of Bircher-Benner apple Müesli (if not used for breakfast).

OR: Bowl of whole grain cereal with prunes, raisins, and fresh milk (if not eaten for breakfast).

OR: Fresh fruit.

Glass of nut-milk * or sesame seed milk (if not eaten for breakfast).

MIDAFTERNOON: Glass of fresh fruit or vegetable juice.*

OR: Cup of herb tea, sweetened with honey.

DINNER: Big bowl of fresh, green vegetable salad.*

2-3 boiled or baked potatoes in jackets.

Prepared vegetable course, if desired: vegetable soup, vegetable stew, beans, peas, eggplant, artichoke, sweet potatoes, etc.

Fresh cottage cheese, preferably homemade.*

1-2 slices of whole grain bread, preferably sour rye bread.*

Fresh butter, slice or two of mild, natural cheese.

Glass of yogurt or homemade soured milk.*

OR: Bowl of Molino,* potato cereal,* millet cereal * or other whole grain cereal with milk, prunes, and/or raisins.

Glass of unpasteurized, fresh milk.

* See Chapter 29 for recipe.

Whole wheat or sour rye bread with butter and natural cheese.

(This alternative only if big bowl of vegetable salad was eaten at lunch. However, vegetable salad could be eaten twice, if desired, both for lunch and for dinner.)

BEDTIME SNACK: Glass of fresh milk with tablespoon of wheat germ and/or tablespoon brewer's yeast and teaspoon of honey.

OR: Cup of your favorite herb tea and one slice of whole grain bread with cheese and butter.

OR: Glass of nut-milk or banana milk shake.*

General Outline Only

The above outline of the diet is only the very general skeleton around which the individual wholesome diet of optimum nutrition should be built.

As the menu suggests, the bulk of your food intake should consist of fresh fruits and vegetables, most of them eaten raw. But you also may prepare some cooked vegetables: soups, stews, steamed vegetables, boiled or baked potatoes and yams, squashes, etc. However, cooked vegetables, delicious as they may be, should be used only sparingly and never *replace* the daily use of fresh, raw vegetables. Fresh, green, leafy vegetables are packed with sun energy, with chlorophyl, enzymes, vitamins, and minerals. They are living and life-giving foods. Fresh, brightly colored vegetables and fruits, particularly green, leafy vegetables, if eaten raw, contain the greatest health potential of all foods.

All available fresh fruits and berries should be used liberally and in their natural state. Exception: citrus fruits. Although

* See Chapter 29 for recipe.

an excellent health food, they should be used sparingly—not more than one orange or one-half of a grapefruit a day, due to the citric acid content of citrus fruits. For the same reason citrus juices should be used with caution: always freshly made, diluted with water, and taken no oftener than twice a week.

Raw fruits also make perfect between-meal snacks.

Avoid all canned, frozen, or preserved fruits and vegetables. Dried fruits, however, can be used liberally: figs, dates, prunes, raisins, etc. They are all excellent foods if sun-dried and unsulfured.

Warnings Concerning Fruits

1. Eat only ripe fruits. Starches in unripe fruits are difficult to digest and can be the cause of digestive disturbances, gas, etc. Moreover, some unripe fruits contain strong acids which could cause decalcification of the body if eaten in considerable amounts. Unfortunately, much of the fruits are picked when they are green to assure easier transportation and longer "shelf life," with the resulting loss of flavor and quality.

2. If you are not able to obtain organically grown fruits and vegetables, wash all your produce very carefully. Apples, peppers, cucumbers, pears, and some other produce are heavily waxed these days. They should be peeled. It is with great reluctance that I give such advice, since most of the minerals and vitamins are usually contained in the peel or immediately below it.

Grains and Seeds

Every kind of whole grain should be used liberally. Whole wheat cereal from freshly ground wheat, with raisins and unpasteurized milk, is a nutrition-packed delicacy. Buy a little electric grinder and grind your own cereals.

One of the few unadulterated foods still available in stores is oatmeal—you know, the rolled type, Quick or Old-Fashioned. You may prepare a hot cereal from them or eat them raw as they come from the package with milk and a little honey and raisins—children just love them that way! Excellent cereals may also be prepared from millet or buckwheat (kasha). Add milk and sprinkle raw wheat germ over it.

Avoid all prepared cereals sold at the supermarket. They are stripped of all the nutritional qualities of the whole grain and are loaded with sugar, preservatives, and chemicals of all kinds. The same could be said of all commercially produced breads, including brown and whole wheat bread. Supermarket bread is loaded with toxic preservatives and conditioners. They take out about 40 vital nutritive factors from the whole wheat grain, add a half-dozen poisonous chemicals, conditioners, and preservatives plus three synthetic vitamins and inorganic iron, and then have the nerve to call it "enriched"!

The only way to get wholesome bread these days is to bake it yourself from freshly ground, organically grown grains. In Chapter 29 you will find recipes for delicious and wholesome whole grain breads.

Beans, peas, and lentils are excellent foods, especially soybeans, which contain twice as much complete high-grade protein as meat does. Use them as often as you can in your favorite dishes.

Use sunflower seeds, sesame seeds, chia seeds, flaxseeds, pumpkin seeds, and every kind of raw nuts—all excellent sources of high-grade proteins, vitamins, and minerals.

Milk

Of all animal proteins, the unpasteurized milk of healthy cows, raised on organic fodder without chemicals and insecticides, is considered best from a biochemical point of view. It contains all the essential amino acids of meat without meat's adverse properties. Yogurt, buttermilk, cultured milk, or other forms of soured milk are excellent and delicious health foods. Powdered skim milk makes a delicious protein- and mineral-rich drink. Use some cheese every day, especially uncreamed cottage cheese.[4] Eat only natural cheese, never so-called processed and pasteurized kinds.

Honey

Honey should be an important part of every optimal diet. Raw, unpasteurized honey is a nutritional wonder of nature, a true gold mine of health-giving and protective nutritive factors. Use honey as a substitute for sugar whenever you need a sweetener.

Vegetable Oils

Avoid hydrogenated and saturated fats: lard, margarines, and animal fats. For a spread use only natural butter. For vegetable salad and cooking use only cold-pressed vegetable oils, available at health food stores. Supermarket varieties of vegetable oil are all chemically treated and their biochemical properties are altered. Cold-pressed olive oil, sunflower oil, safflower oil, soy oil, and flaxseed oil are excellent eating oils, rich in vitamin F, unsaturated fatty acids, and vitamin E. Wheat germ oil, the richest natural source of vitamin E, should be used as a food supplement, especially by persons suffering from arthritis.

Never fry your foods. Boil, broil, or bake, if necessary, but do not fry. Frying changes some of the fatty acids and proteins into a chemical state where they become toxic. Reputable researchers have presented evidence that fried foods may be carcinogenic.

[4] See Chapter 29 for recipe.

Animal Protein

If you absolutely desire to include some animal protein in your diet, use eggs and salt-water fish in preference to meat. Eat eggs no more than twice a week; include fish in your diet only once a week. Remember, the Hunzas, the healthiest people in the world, stay young, virile, and vital and live in perfect health (arthritis is unknown in Hunza) past 100 years of age—and they eat meat not more than once a month. Their diet is a high natural carbohydrate——low animal protein diet as advocated in this book.

Health Destroyers

What not to eat is, perhaps, even more important that *what to eat* when planning a program of vital nutrition.

First and foremost, white sugar and all foods made with it should be totally excluded. Ice cream, candies, sodas, pastries, cakes, cookies, pies, sugared desserts—all must go. The astronomical use of refined white sugar and sugar syrups in the American diet is, to my mind, the greatest health-destroying factor causing the deplorable health condition of the nation.

Coffee, tea, and chocolate drinks, as well as all soft drinks, should be omitted and replaced by wholesome herb drinks and fruit juices. Health food stores carry a wide assortment of delicious herb teas: peppermint, alfalfa, camomile, rose hips, maté, white clover, fenugreek, etc. There you can also acquire a vegetable and fruit juicer, which will make it possible to squeeze fresh juices in your own home.

Salt and all sharp, irritating spices, such as white pepper, mustard, black pepper, etc. must be excluded. When you get accustomed to eating fresh, raw fruits and vegetables you will soon find that they taste delectable even without any seasoning. Even steamed vegetables and baked potatoes taste excellent without salt. This is also true with whole grain breads and cereals. If seasoning for salads or cooked dishes is desired, onions, garlic, dill, sage, watercress, paprika, red chili, and many other herb flavorings will give you a wide variety of choice. Kelp, powdered or granulated, can serve as a salt substitute for a beginner. This seaweed product has a mild, salty taste and could be added to various dishes. Of course, sufferers of arthritis should use a great amount of kelp as a food supplement—it is an extremely beneficial biological therapeutic agent in arthritis.

Food Supplements

The nutritional program outlined in this chapter will provide you with all the known essential food elements as well as all the unknown or undiscovered substances, because this is a diet of *natural* foods, where all the natural food elements are present in proper balance necessary for your optimal health.

There is only one catch. This would be a perfect diet of optimum nutrition provided you can obtain nutritionally superior, organically grown, poison-free fruits, vegetables, and grains. Since for most of us this is impossible and we must use many foods of nutritionally inferior commercial quality, I recommend using certain food supplements. Their purpose is to return to the diet all the nutritive elements destroyed or removed by food manufacturers and processors and to protect us from the poisonous effects of toxic residues. See Chapters 23 and 24 for more details on the question of food supplements.

Note for Persons with Arthritis

The program of vital nutrition outlined above has the greatest potential for optimum health and prevention of disease. It is important to realize, however, that a diet which is perfect for the building of health and prevention of disease is not necessarily the best possible diet for a sick person. Particularly in the case of arthritis, certain specific changes in this general nutritional plan must be made. During the first stages of a therapeutic biological program, for example, all bread and milk should be excluded, with the exception of soured milk and yogurt, sprouted grains, and raw wheat germ. The only form of cheese permitted is homemade cottage cheese. When the patient is well on his way to recovery, whole grain bread and milk and milk products can be gradually added to the diet again. However, a person recovering or recovered from arthritis should always be careful with acid-forming foods: bread, cereals, animal proteins, cheese, etc. It is imperative to continue with the program of vital nutrition long after recovery if lasting results are to be expected. The biological program of treatments establishes favorable conditions in your body for the rebuilding and healing processes to take place. These favorable conditions must be maintained indefinitely in order to assure the continuance of good health and prevent the recurrence of disease.

Important Note

Although it is possible to work out a diet as well as other therapeutic measures in accordance with the program outlined in this book and follow them in your own home, I am conscious of the fact that many patients are not sufficiently informed or are otherwise unable to follow this course with required care.

Therefore I would advise you to put yourself under the care of an understanding physician or practitioner, who is well initiated in nutrition and the principles of biological medicine. Show him this book and let him work out a program of treatments adopted for your specific needs, including diet and/or fasting, which you can then undertake under his expert supervision. Complete peace of mind and trust in the method is imperative for a successful outcome of any and all treatments.

When you undertake your therapeutic program under expert supervision, or in a clinic, the knowledge that your treatment is in professional hands will give you much confidence and peace of mind, which will help your body's healing forces accomplish a fast and permanent recovery.

Chapter 10

Vita Nova—Health Resort on "Swedish Riviera"

Vita Nova is a well-conceived name for one of the most beautifully located biological clinics in Sweden. It is a three-floor villa built on the steep slopes of the Kulla Hills, high over the little, picturesque village of Mölle, and overlooks the lovely and lively Öresund, a narrow strip of sea between Sweden and Denmark. On clear days you can see Sjaelland in Denmark and the village of Gilleleje on the opposite side of the Öresund.

Vita Nova is owned and directed by Dr. Lars-Erik Essén, M.D., specialist in internal medicine and dermatology, the leading pioneer of biological medicine in Sweden.

My visit to Vita Nova was arranged in advance, and I was met at the railway station in Halsingborg, 21 miles away from Mölle. A pleasant half-hour drive along the beautiful coast.

Vita Nova is permitted by the medical government of Sweden to accommodate 30 patients. I found most of them sitting in a huge, sun-drenched dining room which afforded a breathtaking view of the sea. I joined Dr. Essén and his assistant for dinner. As is common in all biological clinics, the table was a festive and colorful sight to behold. It was laden with a wide variety of tasty salads made from fresh, organically grown vegetables, soured milk (buttermilk), cottage cheese, sauerkraut, baked or boiled potatoes, vegetable soup, a protein-rich course made from soybeans, and a wide assortment of other equally nutritious viands.

What Is Biological Medicine?

My first question to Dr. Essén concerned the meaning of the term *biological medicine*. The concept of biological medicine is very exactly defined by Dr. Essén in *Vidi Nova,* a special publication for biological medicine issued by him, which deals with the practical results of applied biological methods. As the foremost representative of biological medicine in Sweden and the leading spirit behind the new and growing movement of progressive doctors following the principles of biological medicine in their practice, Dr. Essén was indeed a man well qualified to answer my question: "What is biological medicine?"

"May I, instead of using dry, scientific definitions, illuminate this with a concrete example," said Dr. Essén. "A doctor is treating a case of infectious disease by the conventional methods. The determining factor for a successful result of this kind of treatment is to identify the kind of bacteria considered responsible for the infection in question. When the intruder is identified, the patient is given a specific chemical or antibiotic drug, which, as a rule, accomplishes the immediate results: the bacteria are destroyed and the patient is free from symptoms.

"After a while, it may happen that the same patient will turn up with a new infection. The diagnosis shows that either it is a question of the same kind of bacteria, which this time, however, is already immune to the specific drug, or there are new bacteria involved. Accordingly, new and more potent drugs are pre-scribed, which bring about immediate results, as far as the fighting bacteria is concerned. But in spite of the "success" of the treatment, the patient's resistance to infection seems to progressively weaken and various complications set in. Now, perhaps, such potent drugs as cortisone—pain-killer and symp-tom-remover—and other highly toxic synthetic drugs enter the picture. The body, already weakened by the disease, must now, in addition, cope with the toxic and damaging side effects of the poisonous drugs.

"Then, one day, we stand by the deathbed surprised and shocked. The patient had received all the correct treatments in accordance with medical science's conventional practices and regulations. The laboratory tests proved that we made no errors! Bacteria samples showed that the bacteria, which our treatment was aimed at, were 'successfully' eradicated. As far as the direct cause of the symptoms was concerned (the bac-teria) our treatment was a complete success. The only problem was the patient died! We succeeded in killing the bacteria, but we failed to save the host organism, where our war on bacteria was so successful. It also could be said that the treatment was successful, but unfortunately, as a result of the treatment and resultant complications, the patient died. Or, 'The operation was successful, but the patient didn't survive.'

"Now, actually, this kind of a result is not so surprising, is it?" continued Dr. Essén. "After all, what did we treat? Our treat-ment was directed at micro-organisms which we considered pathogenic or disease-causing. In the meantime, the biological environment for this micro-organism, the host organism, the living, delicate, sensitive, and easily damaged human body, has actually been completely neglected. The man hardly comes into the picture at all. What we actually treat today are diseases, not the diseased people. The sick body, however, is subject to very different biological laws than those which could be applied in primitive germ war with chemical and antibiotic germ-killers.

"A parallel to this can be seen in today's damage and destruction of life and natural environments as a result of man's indiscriminate use of insecticides and other poisonous chemicals. Is there any intelligent human being who is so naïve as to assume that these poisons will be less devastating to the human body, with its endlessly more intricate and delicate living mechanism? The biological laws of life are quite different from the laws which regulate chemical reactions observed in laboratory tubes. When we fail to see the difference between the two, catastrophic conditions will be the result, and we have to accept the consequences of our unwise actions."

Philosophy of Biological Medicine

"When the biologically oriented physician is confronted with a case of infectious disease his approach and his actions are entirely different. For him, bacteria and viruses which are present in certain infections, are phenomena of secondary interest. He considers them only as symptomatic factors in relation to the host organism (the patient) and his body as a biological environment. All his attention is directed towards the patient. His primary aim is to employ every measure available to increase the power of resistance within the host organism and avoid causing it any damage. The first principle of the art of healing, enunciated already by the Father of Medicine, Hippocrates, 'Primum est nil nocere'—the most important thing of all is that treatment must do no harm—is violated in present-day medical practice more than in any other period of medical history.

"The biologically oriented doctor is aware that with chemical and antibiotic drugs he will always cause damage to the host organism's biological milieu, even though with such treatments he can achieve a temporary effect. Therefore, he avoids to the utmost the use of such drugs in the management of simple and harmless infections. To treat a common cold or a sore throat with, for example, penicillin, for him is a crime against the fundamental rules of health. Instead, his attention is directed to increasing the body's own resistance with all the natural, harmless, biological methods of treatment which are available."

"In your experience, Dr. Essén, are the results of such biological treatments gratifying?" I asked.

"I have had the joy of observing how the body, as a rule, if the general resistance is not too much lowered and if given a chance and proper aid in the form of rest, fasting, wholesome diet, and other biological measures, will by the strength of its own healing power win the battle. And this is not only true in cases of milder infections, but also in cases of very serious diseases. Furthermore—and this is a very essential point—instead of coming out of the disease weakened and debilitated, as is always the case after treatments with chemical drugs, the patient, after biological treatments, comes out strengthened and renewed. It is my observation that biological treatments raise the general resistance of patients and they will, as a rule, become more immune to infections in the future."

Biological Medicine and Arthritis

At this point I wanted to direct Dr. Essén to the specific area of arthritis.

"What is your experience in Vita Nova with arthritis, and how effective are biological methods in the treatment of arthritis?"

"First, we must acknowledge that the conventional, symptomatic drug approach to arthritis has failed to show positive results. Accordingly, patients are left without any alternative. In fact, they are told that there is no alternative.

"But there is an alternative, and sometimes a very effective one, without toxic drugs. This alternative is biological medicine.

"Biological medicine is very adaptable for treating diseases of the rheumatic type because of their systemic and metabolic nature. The biological treatments help restore the normal met-

abolic rate, normalize the functions of the vital organs, assist
the body in elimination of toxic wastes from the system—in
short, rebuild and restore the patient's general health. Although
I believe that dependable scientific conclusions must be made
first after ten years of observation (our clinical work here
started only seven years ago), our preliminary impression is
that biological methods are of supreme importance in the management of arthritis. As you know, we do not specialize in
arthritis only—patients come here with all imaginable ills. But
we have treated a sufficient number of patients with arthritis
already to be able to make the statement that biological treatment will give them a chance either for a complete recovery or,
in most cases, a definite improvement in their condition."

Vita Nova Program of Biological Treatments
for Arthritis

At Vita Nova Dr. Essén makes some important exceptions to
some of the fundamental principles adopted by other major
clinics in Sweden, as follows:

1. Dr. Essén has a general impression, based on practical
experience and existing case histories, that prolonged fasting is
undesirable in the case of rheumatoid arthritis. The same is true
concerning the raw, uncooked diet. Although it is general
observation, including his own personal experience, that fasting
and raw food diets result in an immediate and striking improvement in the condition of the patient, it is all too common that
prolonged, continuous treatment of this kind will very often
result in a change for the worse. The reason for this is that raw
vegetable juices and raw vegetables, as well as fasting, dissolve
the accumulated toxins too fast and thus activate biochemical
changes in the joints to such an extent that the pathologically
affected joints cannot tolerate it, nor can eliminative organs
handle the heavy load of wastes thus thrown into the bloodstream. This invariably leads to deterioration and worsening of

the condition. Raw food therapy and fast therapy, as healing measures, are very powerful curative therapies and should be employed with great caution.

Consequently, Dr. Essén recommends repeated short fasts from three to five days followed by the cleansing diet for the same length of time. The intermediate diet should consist of a mixed raw and cooked vegetable diet, well balanced and individually planned in every case to prevent detoxification from occurring too rapidly.

2. The administration of certain biological preparations (organic medicines) is of very great importance in Dr. Essén's treatments. The biologically oriented physician in Europe has access to a growing line of new biological medicines made from organic and inorganic substances found in nature and prepared in accordance with biological principles. They are never synthetic and never toxic. Several companies in Europe specialize in the production of such remedies. The preparations most used by Dr. Essén are the well-known remedies from Weleda and Wala in Switzerland. These preparations are administered both orally and as subcutaneous injections.

Dr. Essén says, "The therapeutic effect of these kinds of medications lies in the fact that they direct the life-force in the desired direction, stimulate the glands and other vital organs of the body, and accelerate the healing process. They do not alter nor interfere with normal metabolic processes, only support and activate them."

Aside from these two exceptions, Dr. Essén's program is in general similar to what we have described in the previous chapter: lactovegetarian diet, preferably of organically (without sprays and chemical fertilizers) grown products, fasting, enemas, therapeutic baths, physiotherapy, relaxation massage, etc.

In his practice all synthetic and chemical drugs are taboo. He warns, however, that cortisone should not be cut off abruptly. The doses should be reduced gradually until the body has time to adjust to the new situation. He replaces cortisone with biological medicines that stimulate the adrenals, hypophysis, and other endocrine glands.

In addition, he uses large doses of vitamins, particularly vitamin B-12 [1] and large doses of vitamin E (300 milligrams a day), because of its anticollagenotic effect.[2] Furthermore, he uses vitamin C (up to 1,000 milligrams orally or intravenously), also B-complex and C combination. The other remedies to note are pollen preparations, organic mineral supplements, medicinal herbs, biologically prepared elixirs, and *Luvos Heilerde,* a clay preparation which is very effective in absorption and elimination of toxins from the intestinal tract. To the same end he uses various preparations of lactoacid bacteria: *L. acidophilus, L. thermophilus, L. bulgaris.*

The Havoc Played by Cortisone

"The pervading experience at the Vita Nova," says Dr. Essén, "is that patients who have received cortisone treatments prior to coming here respond very slowly to biological treatment. Their response is in direct relation to the extent of their prior treatment with corticosteroids. In some cases damage done by cortisone is so extensive that it is almost impossible to achieve any betterment of the condition.

"Prolonged cortisone treatment results in a complete derangement of the vital physiological functions of the body. Metabolic rate is altered. Hormonal balance is disturbed. The body's own healing and repair mechanisms are put out of order. Perhaps, worst of all, the cortisone-treated patient is subject to mental and emotional disturbances, may be depressed, or have

[1] Vitamin B_{12} neutralizes the ulcer-causing effect of cortisone, regenerates the liver, and counteracts the damaging effect of cortisone, as reported by three Rumanian researchers, Hadnagy, Bird, and Kelemen in *Archives Internationales de Pharmacodynamie et de Therapie,* Sept. 1965.

[2] "Rheumatoid arthritis belongs to the group of diseases called 'collagenoses,' or collagen diseases." Footnote by Dr. Essén.

a negative outlook. It requires a great amount of patience, understanding, and self-discipline, both on the part of the patient as well as on the part of the physician, to go through with the withdrawal of this drug—with, the consequent, often very trying, crises—and the various phases of the biological treatments."

No Magic Wand

Before I left Vita Nova, the picturesque health resort nestled on a hill overlooking the Strait of Öresund, Dr. Lars-Erik Essén gave me these words of advice:

"There is no question that arthritis—if not too advanced—can be cured. Biological methods are the only ones at present which can bring about the cure. *But they are not a magic wand.* Those who expect a quick and easy cure of the take-a-pill-and-you-get-well type, should not even bother to apply. It may take time to effect a complete restoration of health. Every case of arthritis is unique and requires a personalized approach plus specific treatments. Some patients will respond in a few weeks, while in other cases it may take months, even years, to repair all the damage, straighten the joints, and restore complete health. It takes patience and determination, it takes perseverance and burning desire on the part of the patient to get well. But if the will and desire are there—the compensation that will follow is attractive enough to inspire anyone."

Chapter 11

Björkagården—Health Paradise in Sweden

In contrast to the continental Riviera-resort atmosphere of the Vita Nova, Björkagården is located deep in the woods of northern Sweden on the bank of one of the great Swedish rivers —Dala-älven.

Björkagården Health Institute is housed in a centuries-old, authentic timber building originally used as a farmhouse. Ten years ago it was totally rebuilt and enlarged with the original rustic timber style retained. The location is most serene and beautiful. The buildings are surrounded by hundreds of acres of graceful birch and majestic red pine. A breathtaking view over the Dala-älven river, with its pure drinking waters, completes the picture of unspoiled, natural surroundings.

But don't be fooled by the farm-like, rustic exterior. Björkagården is a completely modern clinic with hospital-clean treatment rooms, specially designed bathing rooms, steam houses, etc. It is, perhaps, the most modern and best equipped biological clinic in Sweden at present. At the same time it is very tastefully and artistically decorated with wall-to-wall carpeting throughout, modern Swedish furnishings, and local arts and crafts. It has the pleasant atmosphere of an exclusive private guest home. The maximum capacity of Björkagården is only 18 patients. During my visit it was filled to capacity and had a reservation period of one month's waiting time.

Björkagården is one of the oldest biological clinics in Sweden. Under the same direction of Ingrid Öye-Carlson from its beginning, it was using biological methods of treatment for over 20 years. The clinic does not specialize in rheumatic diseases, as Brandals does—it accepts patients with asthma, skin disorders, high blood pressure, liver and kidney diseases, digestive disorders, etc., in addition to arthritis. However, during the past 20 years Björkagården Institute has treated over 1,000 cases of arthritis.

Here are a few typical cases from the Björkagården files.

The Case of Engineer Karl-Gustav Engberg, Kristinehamn, 46 Years Old

Mr. Engberg was stricken by disease three years ago. It started with liver trouble and jaundice. He also suffered from very bad constipation for years. Eventually his condition was diagnosed as rheumatoid arthritis.

During the following year he received various treatments from several doctors and hospitals: injections, cortisone, even so-called malaria treatment. Various other remedies were tried without any noticeable improvement. Doctors said that his kind of arthritis was a very rare type that would be difficult to cure.

In June, 1964 he came to Björkagården. He could move only with great effort. He was not able to bend his legs or arms. His joints were inflamed, swollen, and stiff.

Mr. Engberg started immediately with a ten day fast. He then went on a special diet for 30 days, followed by a new fast for 21 days. He stayed at the clinic for eight months, alternating fasts with diet periods. Some shorter fasts were pure water fasts. The long fasts consisted mostly of carrot juice and vegetable broth. The final fast lasted 40 days. The unusually long fasts and the length of his stay at the clinic were motivated by his damaged liver and the necessity of reactivating and rebuilding his liver function as a step in the normalizing of his whole metabolism. In his particular case, all milk was excluded from the diet. Raw nuts and seeds were substituted for milk as a protein source.

After eight months Mr. K.-G. Engberg was able to leave the clinic in perfect health. On arriving back at his hometown he visited his doctor and received a complete physical checkup. The surprised doctor could not find any traces of arthritis.

Now Mr. Engberg leads a perfectly normal life. He has resumed his favorite sport activity, pathfinding, and takes part in strenuous training and competitive sports.

The Case of Mrs. F. B., Fränsta, Medelpad, 72 Years Old

Arthritis made Mrs. F. B. a complete invalid. She was also afflicted with chronic anemia. She suffered from arthritis for six years and received all the available medical treatments in various hospitals: drugs, injections, cortisone. Finally she was given up by doctors as incurable and sent to a home for the chronically ill.

In 1950 she came to Björkagården in a wheelchair. She could not move at all; she had to be carried in on a stretcher. She was too weak and too debilitated for fasting. For two months she received a diet of vegetable broth, lots of fresh carrot juice, and a lactovegetarian raw food diet. After two months she started fasting—short three to five day fasts, alternated with periods of eating of the same length. While fasting Mrs. F. B. received only carrot juice.

During her entire stay at Björkagården Mrs. F. B. was under an extensive program of bath therapies: Kuhne-bath, sitz bath, steam bath, etc. She also received wet packs with cider vinegar over her affected joints.

After six months she was able to leave the clinic restored to complete health. To celebrate her return to life she danced a hambo (Swedish polka-type dance) on the day of her departure!

The Case of Mr. Martin Lindgren, Borlänge, 45 Years Old

It started in 1954 with a bad sore throat followed by tonsilitis. He was treated with various drugs. After awhile he started to feel nagging pains, first in his joints and later in his whole body. His doctor in Borlänge diagnosed the condition as rheumatoid arthritis. He had a very high sedimentation rate. The doctor prescribed several drugs, 12 tablets a day, but no cortisone.

In February, 1955 Mr. Lindgren came to Björkagården. He was bedridden with agonizing pains and with badly swollen joints.

His first fast, on pure water, lasted ten days followed by a ten day fast on vegetable and fruit juices. Various baths, massage, vacuum cupping, etc. were included in the program. He fasted a total of 30 days.

After two months in Björkagården Mr. Lindgren could return home without the slightest trace of arthritis. During his stay at the clinic he made several visits to his doctor in Borlänge (nearby city) and each time the doctor reported a steady improvement in his condition, which he attributed to the drugs he prescribed. Mr. Lindgren didn't tell him about his treatments at Björkagården and that he discontinued with drugs long ago. The last examination showed that he was totally free from the disease.

The case was periodically checked—no relapses in over ten years.

I recently contacted Mr. Lindgren myself to find out if his recovery from arthritis was complete and if he had any relapses. This is what he wrote me: "There is nothing wrong with my joints and my general health now. I exercise heavily and feel just great...It is tragic that not all arthritis sufferers have knowledge of the methods which restored my health."

The Case of Mrs. Judith S., Hudiksvall, 60 Years Old

Mrs. Judith S. was afflicted with arthritis for ten years. She received all conventional treatments, such as cortisone, gold injections, aspirin, etc. She stayed at the Nynäshamn Rheumatic Hospital four different times, two to three months each time. She was finally dismissed as a hopeless case. Diagnosis: incurable rheumatoid arthritis.

She came to Björkagården in 1961, badly crippled and deformed with swollen knees and stiff arms. Her whole body was afflicted with arthritis. However, her shoulders and neck were affected the worst. She could not lift her arms.

First, she stayed at the clinic two months during which time she fasted twice, seven and ten days. She returned home improved but not well.

After two months at home she returned to Björkagården and stayed another two months. Again there was considerable improvement. Previously very discouraged and without hope of ever becoming well again, Mrs. Judith S. became encouraged by the improvement in her condition. Now she started to see new hope and the way to a complete recovery. She took a job at the clinic as a helper in the kitchen, doing cleaning, etc., and stayed there for two years! During this time she fasted on several occasions, took all the therapeutic treatments—she even took ice cold baths in the middle of the winter in the nearby Dala-älven river.

After two years Mrs. Judith S. left Björkagården absolutely free from all traces of arthritis. She keeps in periodic contact with the clinic—no relapses.

It Takes Time

The fantastic story of Judith S. above demonstrates that it often takes time and great patience to get well! It takes time to undermine health and create conditions favorable for the development of disease. And it takes time to restore health and create favorable conditions for the repair and rebuilding of damaged joints.

But this story also demonstrates that with perseverance and patience, even for more advanced cases of arthritis where destructive changes are severe, there is a possibility of a complete cure. But, as we said, it may take time, even as long as two years, as in the case of Mrs. Judith S. However, given the chance—and the time—the body sooner or later will respond to biological treatments, and permanent correction of disease and restoration of health will be attained.

The Program of Treatments at the Björkagården Institute

FASTING (3 TO 40 DAYS)

On the first day of fasting only: one hour before enema, two tablespoons of pure castor oil with a glass of water to which juice of half a lemon has been added.

7:00 A.M.	Morning beverage: vegetable broth.*
7:10 A.M.	Dry brush massage.
7:30 A.M.	Massage with Öye-oil and Güsse-shower (hot and cold).

* See Chapter 29 for recipes.

8:00 A.M.	Enema. At Björkagården an enema is given 3 times a day during entire length of fasting.
9:00 A.M.	Glass of juice. Carrot juice * or diluted citrus juice.
10:00 to 11:00 A.M.	Baths: Kuhne-bath (temperature 12-18°C).
	Alternating sitz baths (warm, 15 min., 38°C; cold, ½ minute, 18°C).
	Sauna bath.
11:00 A.M.	Cup of herb tea.*
12:00 A.M.	Vacuum massage, cupping—one hour treatment.
1:00 P.M.	Enema.
1:20 P.M.	Glass of carrot juice or vegetable broth.
1:30 to 3:30 P.M.	Rest.
3:30 P.M.	Specialized baths.
5:00 P.M.	Glass of fruit juice.
7:00 P.M.	Cup of herb tea.
8:30 P.M.	Enema.
9:00 P.M.	Bedtime.

DIET BETWEEN FASTS

Note: Enema is continued twice a day during dieting until the natural rhythm of bowel movements is established.

UPON ARISING:	Excelsior drink.*
7:10 A.M.	Dry brush massage. Vigorous brushing with a stiff bristle or natural fiber brush all over the body for 20 minutes.
7:30 A.M.	Massage with Öye-oil and Gusse-shower.

* See Chapter 29 for recipes.

BREAKFAST: 9:00 A.M.	Bircher-Benner Müesli.*
	Fresh fruit available in season.
	Homemade, unpasteurized, soured milk (yogurt)* with 1 tbsp. wheat germ, 1 tbsp. wheat bran, 1 tbsp. flax meal.
10:00 to 11:00 A.M.	Baths.
11:00 A.M.	Cup of herb tea, sweetened with honey.
11:30 to 12:30 A.M.	Vacuum massage, cupping.
LUNCH: 1:00 P.M.	Big bowl of tossed green vegetable salad * with Golden Oil Dressing.*
	Vegetable soup.
	Boiled or baked potatoes with jackets.
	Prepared vegetable dish: beans, stew, etc.
	Glass of homemade yogurt.
	Homemade whole-grain bread with cheese and butter (not allowed to arthritics).
1:30 to 3:30 P.M.	Rest.
4:00 P.M.	Glass of fruit juice.
DINNER: 5:00 P.M.	The same as lunch or as breakfast.
7:00 P.M.	Cup of herb tea.
9:00 P.M.	Bedtime.

In addition to the above, arthritis patients at Björkagården receive Sano (a special cereal containing mustard seeds), natural vitamin C supplement, a mineral preparation, kelp, and cod liver oil.

* See Chapter 29 for recipes.

Chapter 12

How the Battle with Arthritis Is Won—Greta Friberg Tells Her Story

During my visit to Björkagården Institute I met several patients with arthritis and interviewed some of them. One story is etched into my memory more than any other because it is a dramatic and sad story of human suffering and despair. It is a *circulus vitiosus* of going from doctor to doctor in the hope of finding relief from agonizing pain; staying in hospital after hospital; consuming astronomical amounts of toxic drugs—and only getting worse and worse! But this sad story had a happy ending! Let's hear it from Mrs. Greta Friberg in her own words as follows:

* * * *

"About three years ago, at the age of 42, I started to feel a certain stiffness in my joints, mostly in my hands and shoulders.

95

I didn't pay much attention to it, hoping that it would heal by itself. But the stiffness persisted, on and off, for over a year. Then, in January, 1965, my left hand swelled up and started to ache. I wrapped it in warm wool, which relieved the pain somewhat, but the swelling only continued to increase. Three weeks later my right hand started to swell.

"I went to a doctor, a private practitioner in Borås. The examination showed low blood values (70 per cent) and a high sedimentation rate (50). The doctor sent me to the Borås Hospital. But the hospital was overfilled and I had to wait until April 9, 1965 to enter it. Meantime, the pain in my hands was getting more and more agonizing.

"In the hospital they gave me two different drugs: the first week Bamul, the second week Prednisolone, a hormone preparation. I also received shortwave treatments. After two weeks at the hospital my sedimentation rate improved, and swelling went down a little. I was sent home and asked to return after one week for a checkup. Upon returning I received a new medication, Tanderil, and instructions to take six tablets of it a day. I went back home and continued with Tanderil. It relieved the stiffness in my joints, but after about one week I started to feel sick all over and my face started to swell badly— I looked like a blown-up balloon. I lost my appetite, felt tired all the time, and could not sleep well. One morning I could not get out of bed. I had a fever of over 100° and noticed a rash over my breast. My husband telephoned for a physician, but he couldn't come, so my husband took me to the doctor's office in an automobile. The doctor thought that my condition was quite bad. He said that perhaps the Tanderil was too strong and he advised me to get back home, stay in bed, and not take this drug for a while. I was rather shocked and scared to discover that drugs could be that toxic and that they could make me so ill. I went home and decided to throw away all my drugs. I had a high fever and tried resting in bed, but the fever just continued to climb. I felt sick all over. And, after I discontinued with drugs, the pain in my arms was unbelievable. The slightest move caused the most excruciating pains.

"Now my husband telephoned the hospital in Borås and was advised to take me there immediately. At the hospital I received medication which caused irregular heartbeats and a bad cough. Next day I lost consciousness and remained unconscious for 36 hours. When I woke up, I had a bad nosebleed and my eyes were inflamed. Also my hearing was affected. It was as if I had a very severe cold. My nose and throat were all congested and inflamed, and I could not take in any solid foods. This continued for a whole week. During all this time my fever remained high. Nosebleeding became very bad and they had to burn the inside of my nose to stop the profuse bleeding. After three weeks they put me back on Bamul again. This time I stayed at the hospital a total of seven weeks.

"When I got back home and started using several new prescribed drugs my temperature never did go down. I felt very tired and had to stay in bed most of the time. After four days at home and heavy medication a rash broke out all over my body. I went back to the hospital.

"Now I stayed there for two and a half months. All that time my condition was progressively getting worse. My blood hemoglobin count was now 40. Doctors said that my kidneys were weak and my liver was inflamed. They gave me new drugs, six tablets a day, and sent me home. The hospital doctor sent me to a convalescent home in Hultafors.

"Five weeks at the convalescent home put me on my feet again. I regained some strength and added some weight. Not only did I receive various drugs there, but also shortwave treatments, massage, hot baths, etc. My blood value improved (80 per cent) and stiffness and swelling were relieved somewhat. I returned home able to walk, even though my arms and shoulders were still painful and stiff.

"In January, 1966 my condition took a turn for the worse again. My whole body was swollen. A doctor at the Borås

Hospital said that the swelling was caused by the drugs I was taking. When I stopped taking the drugs the pain in my joints was so unbearable that I could not tolerate it. And now stiffness was spreading all around my body. All the joints were swollen: knees, feet, hips.

"I felt very discouraged and hopeless. They had tried everything and yet I was getting worse. The drugs only made me worse, yet without them my pains were intolerable. I was a nervous wreck and felt very depressed. I wanted to die. There was no way out of the inferno of my agonizing suffering and pain.

"At this point some friends told me of the Björkagården Institute. My husband felt that perhaps it was worth trying. I did not reflect one way or another—I could hardly get worse, so I had nothing to lose.

"I came here on March 18, 1966. Immediately I was put on a 17 day fast. It wasn't easy, I must admit. My nerves were bad, I was worried and irritable. But after 17 days of fasting, to my surprise, I felt a fantastic improvement! The pain was all but gone (and without drugs, because all my drugs were taken away from me the day I arrived) and my joints regained some mobility. Of course, during the fast, which consisted of fresh juices and vegetable broths, I received all the usual treatments here: baths, vacuum massage, cupping, etc. I returned home in better condition than I had experienced in many years.

"After one week home I returned here to continue my treatments. I fasted one week on water; then I went on a special diet for four weeks. After that I fasted one more week on juices. I went home for a week, much improved, but still felt some stiffness in the joints, especially my knees and hips. Later, I returned here on June 5 to complete my treatments, and have been here now for six weeks. I fasted on juices for 21 days. Now I am on my special diet again.

"The last long fast did wonders for me! Now I am completely free from pain. The joints are almost normal; no swelling, just a slight stiffness occasionally. But I know that a couple weeks more and I will be completely cured. I feel like a new person. I swim in the river every day and take long walks. I am so grateful! I plan to stay here until the 15th of August, but I feel so great already that I could go home today!"

* * * *

This is the inspiring story of Mrs. Greta Friberg in her own words. It is a true story of the failure of the conventional drug approach to solve the problem of arthritis and the triumph of simple, natural biological methods in conquering disease and restoring health.

I had to leave Björkagården the following morning and continue my journey to the other Swedish clinics I was scheduled to visit. I could not resist taking an early morning walk in the beautiful woods which surround the clinic. I met Mrs. Friberg on the trail a couple of miles from the house, in the deep, misty woods. It was seven o'clock in the cool, Swedish summer morning. Dressed in a light "training overall" (flannel slacks and jacket of a sweat shirt type) she was returning from her three mile morning routine. Her cheeks were rosy, she looked exhilarated, happy, and full of zest.

"It is so wonderful to be able to walk again like everybody else," she exclaimed when she saw me approaching. "I wasn't able to do this for many years. This last fast just did wonders for me. Now I know that I am finally winning the battle!"

Chapter 13

The Fast Recovery of Guldi Deiber

Here is another remarkable case from the files of the Björkagården Institute.[1]

It all started during the hot summer of 1957. Mrs. Guldi Deiber started to feel a dull pain in her muscles. She hoped that it was something that would pass. But the pain didn't go away. Instead it became worse with every new day. Then, a few weeks later, she noticed that the joints of her arms and legs started to swell.

She recalled that she had similar symptoms about 20 years ago, but then the pain gradually disappeared. This time she didn't seem to be able to shake it off; it only became worse each week. Her knees and hips were particularly painful.

Mrs. Deiber went to a doctor. He prescribed a drug. Several

[1] *Tidskrift för Hälsa*, December 1963. Used by permission.

weeks of medication didn't help. Then she visited a new doctor, he prescribed new drugs and so on—an endless cycle of visits from doctor to doctor, from one hospital to another hospital, from one toxic drug to another. When a drug caused unpleasant side effects, she was prescribed a new drug to mask the symptoms caused by the previous drug. This continued for four years. Although some of the drugs she received were able to dull temporarily her unbearable pains, her condition was growing worse.

The most horrifying experience she had with powerful drugs occurred in 1962. Her doctor prescribed a new and controversial drug called Imagon. Its effect on pain was remarkable. Pain disappeared as if by magic and happy Mrs. Deiber continued with the drug from October, 1962 to April, 1963. At this time she noticed that her eyesight was becoming impaired. Everything began to look hazy to her. She hurried to the doctor who had prescribed Imagon.

"Oh, it hurt your eyes already," was the doctor's comment.

Damaged eyesight was the price Mrs. Deiber paid for temporary relief from pain!

Now she was referred to an eye specialist and had to go to this doctor three times a month during the summer of 1963. When the doctor finally prescribed cortisone, she became alarmed and reluctant to use such powerful drugs again—after all, she already had a very bad experience with drugs before!

A good friend suggested that she try wheat germ oil for her eyes. Mrs. Deiber had already taken six cortisone tablets by that time. She discontinued using the drug and started taking six capsules of wheat germ oil each day instead, reduced later to four capsules a day. At the same time she continued to visit her eye specialist every ten days. After a few weeks on wheat germ oil the doctor noticed an improvement in her eye condition. Further improvement was registered with each visit to the doctor.

Meanwhile, her arthritis was becoming more and more unbearable. Violent pains in her joints continued day and night; and now she didn't dare use any more pain-killing drugs. She had difficulty raising herself up from a chair without help. In the morning, her whole body was stiff and the slightest movement caused piercing pains.

At this time she met an old friend who had suffered from arthritis who just returned from the Björkagården Clinic. She saw how much better her friend felt—the woman could now do all her housework with ease, she took long walks, etc. Should she try? She didn't know what else to do. Doctors had tried everything for four years without success. She decided to try the "nature cure" at the Björkagården Institute.

Mrs. Guldi Deiber came to Björkagården Clinic on September 13, 1963. She was tired and very depressed. In addition to excruciating pains in all her joints she had a frightful chronic headache. She felt so debilitated that she had to stay in bed much of the time.

She stayed at the clinic three weeks. The first week she was on a special diet. It was the usual diet of the clinic—but far different from the "usual" diet Mrs. Deiber was accustomed to at home. No coffee and pastry, to which Mrs. Deiber was so addicted! Instead, it was vegetable broth with flaxseed for the morning beverage; yogurt and fresh fruits for breakfast; or a choice of several cereals: brown rice, potato cereal,[2] whole grain cereal, Molino.[2] Lunch consisted of a big bowl of vegetable salad with oil dressing. Dinner was the same as breakfast. In between meals she drank fresh juices and herb teas.

After one week she felt better, but tiredness and pain remained. The next phase of her treatment was fasting. She fasted five days on juices and vegetable broths. After fasting

[2] See Chapter 29 for recipes.

she continued on the same lactovegetarian diet prescribed the
week before her fast.

The results of the three week stay at Björkagården could be
summed up like this:

Her condition was improving steadily during all three weeks.
Particularly during the fast she felt a great improvement. At
the time she left the clinic she was completely free from pain
and felt better than any other time during the past four years.
The swelling in her joints disappeared. In addition to the disappearance of the arthritis symptoms she noticed other im-
provements in her health. She had suffered from sciatic nerve
trouble in both legs, which now totally disappeared. She lost
six pounds. Her sedimentation rate went down from 33 to 15.
Her blood pressure, although not too high previously, went
down from 130 to 115.

Happy and healthy Mrs. Deiber returned to her home full
of enthusiasm for the new, healthful way of life she had found
at the Björkagården Institute.

"Did you have any difficulties adapting yourself to the diet
and the treatments at the clinic?" I asked her.

"No, actually it was not difficult at all. But the right attitude
is important. You just can't passively let them treat you with a
doubtful wait-and-see-what-happens attitude. When I decided
to try this method I also decided then and there to do it whole-
heartedly and cooperate completely. I was fortunate to have
enthusiastic support and encouragement from my husband
Now, we both are sold on this new way of life. We will continue
with lactovegetarian health foods at home. Actually, my husband always wanted to try health foods, but we didn't know
how to go about it.

"Now I have a new and clearer insight into the problems of
health and disease. I know that most diseases are of our own
making. I will continue with the new way of life. To go back to
the old living habits would mean inviting disease back to my
door," concluded happy Mrs. Guldi Deiber, who not only re-

covered from a bad case of arthritis but has found a new, healthier, happier way of life!

This was in September of 1963. Three years later, in September of 1966, I asked Mrs. Deiber if her cure was permanent. She replied that she felt fine and that her arthritis had not recurred since she left the clinic.

Chapter 14

Alfta Clinic—The Center for Biological Medical Research in Northern Sweden

One of the most dedicated pioneers of biological medicine in Sweden is Dr. Jern Hamberg, M.D. Although a very young looking man—I didn't ask his age but he looked to me to be in his late thirties—Dr. Hamberg has had nearly 20 years of experience in biological medicine.

Recently he has opened a private clinic in Alfta, near Bollnäs, in Norrland.

At the time of my visit there, July, 1966, the clinic was closed due to a complete rebuilding and face-lifting. It was to reopen on the 15th of September, modernized and equipped with the latest facilities for biological treatments.

The location of the clinic is extremely beautiful. Just a mile or so away from the town of Alfta, it is situated on a hill surrounded by beautiful and graceful white birches. The nearby river affords bathing in the summer. Several skiing hills, complete with electric elevator and other features, supply a wonderful opportunity to engage in winter sports. Hundreds of acres of unspoiled woods and meadows provide plenty of opportunities to take hikes and tranquilizing walks!

All of this, of course, is not a coincidental occurrence. During our conversation Dr. Hamberg stressed time after time the great importance of exercise and a tranquil, positive mental attitude. He considers physical activity and peace of mind to be the two major therapeutics of biological medicine. Alfta Clinic affords excellent opportunities for these two therapies.

Mental Attitude of Utmost Importance

"Dr. Hamberg," I asked, "conventional medical treatments have failed to show any lasting curative results in arthritis; does biological medicine present a better alternative to the problems of arthritis? Is there a cure for arthritis?"

"Yes, there is a cure for arthritis. Not the quick and easy one. If the patient wants to accept a narrow, steep, and stony path instead of a wide and smooth road; if he has the will and determination to work and fight for his health; if he starts biological treatments in the early stages of the disease—then he will triumph over arthritis.

"Arthritis is a very capricious disease. No two cases are identical. Almost every case requires an individual approach. Some cases respond very quickly, others seem to be completely incurable. But even in bad cases biological treatments will arrest further development of the disease.

"In some cases it may take a long time to bring about a cure. The patient has to be prepared for bad setbacks and patience-trying reactions. He must have perseverance to go through a series of repeated fasts. In other words, he must be willing and prepared for a long battle. The mental attitude of the patient is, therefore, of the utmost importance. We don't cure the patients —they cure themselves with our help. But if they don't value their good health enough to sacrifice, endure, and foresake anything—then they will have no chance. In my experience, the patients who really want to get their health back will ultimately achieve their desire."

Exercise Is Important

"Various physiotherapeutic treatments and exercises form an extremely important part of our program. Arthritics should have as much exercise as possible: long walks, calisthenics, bicycle rides, etc. Therapeutic baths are also essential, particularly sweat baths and hot and cold alternating baths."

Lactovegetarian Diet

"However, the determining biological measures in treatment of arthritis are fasting and proper diet. Patients too weak to fast we put on a special diet to build up their strength. All patients strong enough to fast we immediately put on a fresh juice fast lasting seven to 17 days. After that, the patient lives on a lactovegetarian diet.

"The important part of our work is to instruct patients in the proper way of eating and teach them other health-promoting factors. Then, after fasting, they can return to their homes and practice what they have learned here. After two to three months they can return for another fasting and treatment period. This way, bit by bit, we try to put pieces together and finally restore all bodily functions to normal."

Results of Biological Research

Dr. Hamberg's Clinic, in association with other biologically oriented doctors, is presently engaged in a long-range research project directed at the evaluation of biological methods of treatment for arthritis. This is strictly scientific research which includes both conventional and biological methods of treatment for comparative values. The results of this research are not available as yet.

"However, my experience so far points out the fact that biological methods are, indeed, superior in management of most degenerative diseases, including arthritis," concludes Dr. Hamberg.

"Physician, Heal Thyself ..."

The biblical proverb: "Physician, heal thyself—then you will be able to heal the sick," is more timely at the present time than it was in any other period of medical history.

It is a well-known fact that members of the medical profession as a whole do not present very convincing examples of good health for their patients. Statistics show that their death rate due to heart conditions and other "diseases of civilization" is way up at the top, compared with other professional groups.

My impression of the many biologically oriented doctors and practitioners I met is quite different from what their colleagues in allopathic medicine are famous for. The majority of them are shining examples of the correctness of their way of life. Biological doctors themselves are the best advertisements of the "product" they sell—good health. Not only do they teach others a new and better way of life, but they "practice what they preach," and are (with their own example of what the right way of living can do) inspiring their patients to adopt a better, healthier way of life.

Dr. Jern Hamberg is a good example of the great physician which the biblical proverb speaks of. He lives exactly what he preaches and has, therefore, a deep understanding of what perfect health is and how it can be attained. He is passionately dedicated to help his fellowman. He is humble, understanding, sincere, unselfish, and is motivated by true Christian ideals to give help to the sick and afflicted Such qualities in a doctor are bound to inspire his patients and help them in their recovery.

Chapter 15

Dr. Karl-Otto Aly—Enthusiastic Exponent of Biological Medicine

I have met and talked with many Swedish medical doctors who are, what I termed "biologically oriented," or who acknowledge the value of biological methods of treatment and employ them in their practice. One of the most dedicated and enthusiastic exponents of biological medicine is Dr. Karl-Otto Aly, M.D.

When I met Dr. Aly he had just returned from an extensive lecture tour of the United States. He gave dozens of lectures in cities across the country. The program was organized under the auspices of the National Health Federation. Dr. Aly informed the American public of the significance of the Swedish Health Movement, as pioneered by Are Waerland, and of the role of biological medicine in the prophylactic and therapeutic application of this health program.

We were sitting in the beautiful garden of Brandals Health Clinic overlooking the Baltic Sea, and our conversation, naturally, was centered around arthritis.

"Chronic arthritis or rheumatoid arthritis is one of the most difficult and crippling diseases we have in Sweden," stated Dr. Aly. It is estimated that over one-quarter of a million people are afflicted with it here. We spend millions of crowns every year on the medical care of arthritis sufferers, but in spite of all the new drugs, better diagnostic methods, and better hospitals the mystery of arthritis still remains unsolved. Conventional treatments give no lasting improvement and the disease only progresses to a stage where the patient will be more and more incapacitated.

"This pessimistic outlook, however, is not shared by all medical practitioners. As you have seen, we now have several centers in Sweden which are employing new approaches to combat the problem of arthritis. In the Brandals Clinic, as well as in other similar clinics throughout Sweden, biological treatments have been tried with very encouraging results. Our general experience is that biological methods of treatment do indeed affect the disease in a favorable direction and in many cases accomplish a complete cure.

"Actually, biological medicine is better developed and more widely practiced in Germany and Switzerland where there are dozens of huge clinics which employ biological methods of treatment. Here in Sweden we are slowly moving towards this direction, although the official medical body is still skeptical in regard to its value. But then, official medicine was always conservative and accepted virtually every new major medical discovery only after initial skepticism and stubborn resistance."

"Dr. Aly, would you give me, in a nutshell of course, your theory of the causes of arthritis and the biological program of treatments you would advocate?" I asked.

Causes of Arthritis

"Well, when it comes to the exact causes, it is not easy to pinpoint them. There are many theories of course. The most popular explanation is that arthritis is caused by metabolic disturbance. Of course, metabolic disturbance is a very general term. Some researchers feel that the main culprit is a disturbed balance in the intestinal bacterial flora. Normally, the permeability of intestinal walls is limited to beneficial substances. In the case of impaired permeability, due to a bacterial imbalance in the intestines and damage to the mucous membranes of the intestinal walls brought about by toxins, toxic substances also penetrate through the intestinal walls. This results in accumulation of toxins in the whole organism, especially in the connective tissues around the joints, which is one of the leading causes of arthritis. Although the *exact* mechanics of the development of arthritis cannot be pinpointed with certainty, it can, nevertheless, be said that metabolic disturbance and accumulation of toxic substances (metabolites) in the joints are the main causative factors in the onset of arthritis. The exact mechanics, perhaps, will never be found out. Instead, it is of great importance to know what causes the metabolic disturbance which leads to arthritis. All experience and observations—empirical, statistical, and clinical—point out that the causes for degenerative pathological changes leading to arthritis are found in the general deterioration and breakdown of man's resistance. This degeneration is due to his unhealthy, disease-producing, 'civilized' way of life characterized by: lack of exercise, devitalized diet, poisonous environment, smoking, poisonous drugs, emotional and physical stress, etc. Of these, faulty nutrition is, perhaps, the most significant health-destroying factor.

"Now, due to these abuses, the eliminative and protective system of the body breaks down. Toxins and metabolic wastes remain in the organism and are deposited in the tissues, including the joints. Inflammation of the joints is the body's defensive reaction against toxins and seems to be allergic in nature. This results in pain and swelling. The final step is decalcification of the bones, which is the result of diminished use of the joints. At the same time, the damaged tissues or destroyed surfaces of the joints are repaired or replaced by calcification (deposits of calcium). This calcification eventually leads to total fusion of the joints and consequent progressive immobilization and characteristic arthritic deformations."

The Direction of Treatment

"Naturally, effective biological treatment should be directed towards elimination of the underlying causes which lead to pathological changes. The general health must be rebuilt and resistance strengthened. Through proper diet and fasts the functions of protective and eliminative organs of the body should be restored. But diet and fast are not enough. The effective biological program should include a thorough examination for possible foci of infections—teeth, tonsils, lungs, etc., and various physiotherapeutic treatments—baths, heat applications, packs, massage, an effective program of exercises, etc."

Diet

"The diet which is most conducive to restoration of health for an arthritic patient, is the so-called lactovegetarian diet which includes a predominance of fresh raw fruits, vegetables, and whole grains. It should be a *low-protein* diet, with exclusion of meat and fish. Also white sugar, white flour, and all products made from them should be eliminated. Even milk and milk products should be eliminated in the beginning of the treatment, but they can be gradually incorporated into the diet later, when health is restored.

"Such a diet will not only help to restore health, but also it will sustain health in the future and prevent degenerative diseases, including arthritis," concludes Dr. Aly.

Chapter 16

More Actual Case Histories of Cures

In the previous chapters I have presented about a dozen actual cases of arthritis which were cured by biological therapies in Swedish clinics. The majority of them were severe cases of rheumatoid arthritis which received all the conventional remedies and therapies from medical doctors and hospitals and were given up as hopeless, incurable cases. As I have mentioned before, these are just a few examples taken from the thousands of cases of arthritis treated in Swedish biological clinics. I have interviewed many of these patients personally. Some cases are taken from the files of *Tidskrift för Hälsa,* and are used by permission. All of the cases have been authenticated and checked. In cases which were not interviewed personally, I sent questionnaires to the patients and asked for their signed statements. I also got permission to describe their cases and use their names in my book. The reported cases and facts are taken directly from the above-mentioned sources. All this material, together with many photographs of the patients and their original handwritten statements of the accomplished cures, are in my files and are available to all concerned for investigation and study.

Here, briefly, are a few more actual cases of arthritis having been healed, as follows:

Mr. G. A., 31, Solna, Sweden

In the winter of 1950-51 Mr. G. A. was stricken with rheumatic fever. He was only 16 years old at the time. Then in 1957 he had a case of a very bad and persistent cold with severe complications, including inflammation of the ligaments in his feet. In 1958 the pain spread to the neck, shoulders, and back. He received various medications, but without much results. Finally he was referred to the St. Göran Hospital in Stockholm where various tests were made. From there he was sent to the Rheumatic Department of the famous Karolinska Institute.

He stayed at the Karolinska three months. In addition to the various drugs, he received hot bath treatments and corrective exercises. He improved somewhat and was now able to walk "a little." After his return from the hospital he became worse again, in spite of several drugs he was taking, including cortisone. His doctors finally classified him as a "chronic case" and recommended rehabilitation and changing his job as a printer, since he could not stand on his feet. In 1961 he finished his rehabilitation course and started his work as a camera technician.

In 1963 his condition took a turn for the worse. It became more and more difficult for him to get to his job and back home again. He could not walk and the slightest movements resulted in unendurable pain. Even cortisone didn't help anymore. Doctors diagnosed his case as incurable. Confinement in a wheelchair for the rest of his life was all he could look forward to.

But, as they say, "The night is always darkest just before the dawn." Friends brought him a health magazine where biological therapies were described. He decided to give them a try.

He went to the Brandals Clinic in December, 1963. After three weeks of fasting and other biological therapies, plus a few weeks of a special diet, Mr. G. A. was completely free from pain and could walk and move with no apparent difficulty without the aid of crutches.

"The difference is just like night and day," said Mr. G. A. "I still have difficulty believing that I can get up in the morning and stand on my feet without pain and without the need of supporting myself."

Mrs. E. L., 47, Älgarås, Sweden

Mrs. E. L. noticed the first symptoms of arthritis in 1956. She felt a dull pain and stiffness in her hands. The pain spread to the other joints: elbows, shoulders, legs, and feet. Eventually the whole body was affected and the pain became more and more intense.

She was referred by her doctor to the Lidköping Hospital. There she received x-ray treatments plus some drugs. In 1957 her doctor prescribed cortisone. In 1958 she was treated with gold injections at the Mariestad Hospital which resulted in slight improvement in her knees. In 1961 she was again treated with gold injections and other drugs in Nynäshamn Hospital but without any improvement. She stayed at the hospital for two months.

During all these years of conventional treatments with drugs, x-rays, cortisone, and gold injections her condition was gradually getting worse. Her joints were badly deformed and the pain became more and more unbearable.

Finally, in 1962, Mrs. E. L. came to the Björkagården Institute. She stayed there six weeks and fasted five days on juices. She felt great improvement; pain and stiffness disappeared. In 1963 she returned for six more weeks and this time she fasted ten days.

After a second visit to Björkagården her arthritis was all but gone. Pain disappeared and joints became flexible and mobile. She continued with the lactovegetarian diet in her home, and reported to me in August, 1966 that she felt great and had no recurrence.

Mrs. I. B., 39, Borlänge, Sweden

Mrs. I. B. was stricken with arthritis at the age of 22. First, she noticed a swelling in the joints and then later stiffness and pain. She was treated with various drugs. Her condition was steadily getting worse until 1958 when she had to go to a hospital in Halmstad. She made several hospital visits during 1958-63. In spite of these treatments and several drugs she didn't notice any improvement in her condition.

In 1964 she came to Björkagården Institute. She stayed there three weeks and fasted three times. After three weeks of intensive biological treatments and fasts her arthritis was completely gone. In answer to my inquiry as to the results of her treatments in Björkagården and the permanency of her cure, Mrs. I. B. wrote, in September, 1966:

"Results were fantastic. No arthritis left . . . No relapses!"

Mr. S. K., 40, Stockholm

The first symptoms of arthritis appeared in 1952. The contributing cause: a stubborn case of chronic tonsilitis. The pain in his joints continued on and off for several years. A visit to a doctor resulted in the removal of his tonsils. But the pain and the stiffness in the joints didn't disappear. With the passing years it only seemed to become worse.

Finally, he was referred to the Sodersjukhuset in Stockholm. There he was treated with gold injections.

In 1957 he started with cortisone. At first he felt great improvement. Then the pain and the stiffness returned. In 1959 he was sent to the Karolinska Institute and stayed there three months—no improvement.

During 1961 and 1962 he was trying to keep going with the help of cortisone—16 milligrams a day, a very heavy dose. In addition to cortisone he was taking various other drugs, including sulfa drugs and salicylates. He estimates that during a period of six years he had consumed 25,000 aspirin tablets! All these drugs didn't help his condition at all. His arthritis was getting progressively worse with aggravated and intensified pain and stiffness.

In 1963 Mr. S. K. went to Brandals Clinic. Treatments at Brandal started with the traditional fast. He fasted for 20 days and felt better and better with each day of fasting. After the first week all pain and stiffness disappeared. For the first time in many years he could clench his hands together. After 20 days of fasting, consequent special diet, and other biological treatments his long battle with arthritis was finally won.

Miss S. N., 39, Boden, Sweden

Miss S. N. is a practical nurse. At the age of 18 she started to feel pain in both her feet. Eventually pain spread to other parts of the body. Then swelling of the joints appeared, and consequent stiffness accompanied it. Doctors were using all the conventional therapies on her, including a long list of drugs: ACTH, cortisone, Imagon, Tanderil, Magnecyl, etc. In addition, she stayed several times, for many weeks at a time, at the Rheumatic Clinic of Boden Hospital and received all the orthodox treatments there. Heavy doses of drugs killed the pain somewhat, but as soon as she stopped taking them the pain recurred with even more intensity than before.

In 1964 she came to Björkagården Clinic. There she fasted
for ten days. She left the clinic in much better condition but
not completely cured. She returned again in 1965 and one
last time in 1966 for three weeks of therapy. In September, 1966
Miss S. N. wrote to me:

"I cannot say that I am completely cured as yet. But I feel
so much better and I am most grateful that I can now live
without pain and without drugs. I didn't take one single tablet
since 1963!"

Mrs. K. A., 56, Gothenburg

Mrs. K. A.'s arthritis was diagnosed in 1963. It started with
the classic symptoms of dull pain in the joints followed by
swelling. Pain became more and more severe with every passing
week.

For the next two years Mrs. K. A. visited several doctors and
stayed in various hospitals where she received the usual conventional drug treatments. She stayed at the Gothenburg
Hospital and at the Lidköping Hospital. None of the conventional treatments brought an improvement or alleviation of her
suffering.

In 1965 she came to Björkagården Institute and stayed there
two weeks, fasting for seven days. When she came to Björkagården she could walk only with great difficulty. She returned
home much improved, but not completely cured. In 1966 she
returned to the clinic. This time she stayed three weeks and
fasted ten days. After the second visit her arthritis was all gone,
pain and stiffness disappeared, and she could return home in
perfect health.

Mrs. A. A., Harbonäs, Sweden

One of the most moving and inspiring stories of victory
over destructive and crippling disease is the case of Mrs. A. A.

Mrs. A. A.'s family lived happily on a ranch and everything was well until Mrs. A. A. was suddenly stricken with a severe case of rheumatoid arthritis. She went the usual round of visits to doctors and hospitals and received all the conventional treatments—all to no avail. Her disease seemed to defy every drug and every therapy. She was rapidly becoming more and more crippled until she was totally invalided and bedridden. She could not take care of her seven small children and her husband. She wasn't able to look after the home and milk and feed her cows. Finally the doctors and the local health authorities decided to send her to an institution for chronic invalids. The children were to be sent to various foster parents in the area. Thus a once happy family was to be broken up and dispersed.

But Mrs. A. A. had a lucky break. She read in a magazine about Brandals Clinic and the successful arthritis cures accomplished there. This magazine article saved her from living the rest of her days as a helpless invalid and kept her family and children together. She came to Brandal on January 20, 1956 as a bedridden invalid. She fasted 20 days and received all the other biological treatments. After 26 days at Brandal on February 16, 1956 she was able to return to her home in perfect health. She could walk and move without pain and stiffness.

When I heard this story and consulted the records at Brandal, I asked Mrs. Nissen to personally check this case and confirm the permanency of the cure. On July 17, 1966, ten years after her successful arthritis cure, we telephoned Mrs. A. A. directly from the clinic. Her daughter answered the telephone. Here is the conversation that followed:

"Is your mother home?"

"Yes, she is out in the field loading hay on the truck."

"Would you, please, call her in? This is Mrs. Nissen from Brandal speaking."

A few minutes later Mrs. A. A. was on the line.

"Hello, dear A., how are you? How is your arthritis and how are your seven children?"

"What arthritis? I didn't have any feeling of it since I left Brandal ten years ago. I am feeling fine, working every day doing heavy farm labor and taking good care of all my children. Except that there are eight of them now! The youngest is six years old."

Mr. D. S., 55, Gislaved, Sweden

Time: winter 1962. Scene: skiing track for competitive sports in Sweden. Result: seven miles in 50 minutes.

Well, those of you who are authorities on skiing may say that this is not so remarkable. If, however, you were familiar with all of the circumstances involved you might change your mind. The man who accomplished the above feat was 51 years old at the time and, in addition, just a few years earlier was not only unable to ski, or run, or walk, but was not even able to sit up in a wheelchair—he was totally incapacitated by arthritis and permanently bedridden, unable to move at all!

Mr. D. S. was stricken by the disease quite unexpectedly. As is often the case with rheumatoid arthritis, it came in like a lion, spread havoc in his joints, and caused fearful pains and destruction. He visited several doctors and stayed at the most famous conventional arthritis clinics in Sweden. Cortisone, gold injections, and an endless line of other drugs were tried on him without bringing about any betterment in his condition. Finally, he had to depend on crutches. But eventually even crutches had to be discarded, and he became permanently beridden. The catastrophe was total. Doctors gave up his case and diagnosed him as a chronic, incurable invalid! Day and night he suffered from the most torturous pains. Needless to say, his spirits were low and he lost all hope of ever being restored to health again.

Some of his friends heard of someone who recovered from arthritis at Brandals Clinic. Would he try? Why not, what could he lose? Mr. D. S. telephoned Alma Nissen and made an appointment.

Treatments at Brandal started with a fast. But Mr. D. S. was depressed and uncooperative. He didn't have much faith in "nature cure." After all, the best medical authorities in the country tried to help him and gave up. He didn't want to fast, didn't want to eat health foods. He regretted that he came there. But Mrs. Nissen finally persuaded him to try.

On the seventh day of fasting Mr. D. S. was able to get up from his bed without help. After nine days he was able to move around without much effort or pain. He returned home and continued with the diet suggested at the clinic. A bad relapse occurred within a few weeks of his departure from the clinic, but a short fast undertaken at his own home quickly restored health and the pain disappeared again. He continued with the lactovegetarian diet religiously and is now completely free of all traces of arthritis which previously had chained him to his bed as a totally incapacitated invalid.

"Fasting and a vegetarian raw food diet have saved my life," says happy and grateful D. S.

Part Two

QUESTIONS AND ANSWERS CONCERNING ARTHRITIS

Chapter 17

How Healing by Fasting Can Be Undertaken at Home

Of all the various therapeutic measures employed by biological medicine in treatment of arthritis fasting is, perhaps, singularly *the most important one.*

Fasting has been used in treating arthritis for centuries, mostly in Europe, but also on this continent. The big difference is that in the United States the majority of doctors who employ fasting in their practice usually advocate a complete or water fast, while European, biologically oriented doctors employ mostly juice fasts.

Although fasting is without a doubt one of the safest therapeutic agents known to medicine,[1] in the minds of the uninitiated and uninformed it is often associated with fear of the possibility of doing harm to the body. This is quite understand-

[1] Arnold De Vries, *Therapeutic Fasting,* Chandler Book Co., Los Angeles, 1963.

131

able, considering that the average man has the impression that complete abstinence from food just for a couple of weeks would result in death. The truth is that man can live without food for months. In fact, man can kill himself by overeating in a shorter time than by fasting.[2] There are recorded cases of fasting up to 90 days on water and up to 249 days on juices and liquids. In recent tests at Stobhill General Hospital, in Glasgow, Scotland, a 54-year-old woman was put on a liquid fast and lost 74 of her 262 pounds *along with a painful arthritic knee condition,* during a fast of 249 days![2] Although therapeutic fasting usually is of no longer duration than 40 days, the great majority of fasts in European clinics are ten to 20 days long.

Although liquid fasting is not a dangerous measure and could be safely undertaken without supervision at home, I would advise that the average patient, who does not have a thorough understanding and insight into all the details and various phases of fasting, should *not* undertake it on his own, but only under expert supervision. This will assure him of peace of mind which is imperative for the successful outcome of any therapeutic measure.

In Sweden, fasting is a national sport. Thousands of healthy young and old, men and women members of the national health organization, Hälsofrämjandet (Health-promotion, Inc.), fast for a week or two every year. Regular short fasts are considered an effective way to cleanse the body of wastes, build up resistance and physical stamina, and prevent diseases. Contrary to popular belief, you don't get weakened or depleted by fasting. On the contrary, fasting will strengthen the body in many ways. The stomach and digestive tract will receive a rest and will be strengthened by fasting. Actually, the total regeneration and rejuvenation of all functions of the body is the objective which induces thousands of Swedes to fast. These fasts are done on

[2] *Lancet,* British Medical Journal, October, 1966.

their own, in their own homes, without supervision of doctors. But then again, these Swedes are experts in fasting; they are well informed and acquainted with the mechanics and philosophy of fasting.

Just to show you how safe fasting actually is, I like to refer to two famous fast-hikes, which were performed in Sweden in recent years under the direction of Dr. Lennart Edrén, world famous authority on fasting. First, 11 Swedish health enthusiasts walked from Gothenburg to Stockholm (over 300 miles) in ten days. During that time they fasted—did not consume any foods at all, only plain water. A couple of years later about 20 persons repeated the hike under tight scientific control. During the whole hike, and for an extended period after it, various medical tests of their condition were made: blood count, blood sugar tests, heart tests, pulse, physical endurance tests, etc. All tests showed that in spite of the unusual stress of the combined fasting and strenuous hike, all participants were in perfect health and did not suffer any damage of any kind. However, quite the contrary was later found to be true because of the discovery that some of the participants were freed from various ailments they suffered before the fast-hike began.

At the time of my last visit to Sweden in July of 1966, Dr. Edrén himself had already fasted a total of 45 days so far that year. At 50 he is a picture of youthful vitality and health, and he is regularly fasting to keep his superior health condition at an optimum level.

Americans Unaware of Fasting Benefits

Unfortunately, in the United States, the average physician, as well as the average layman, are completely unaware of fasting and its extraordinary prophylactic and therapeutic properties. Perhaps the idea of "caring for your own health" or do-it-yourself health measures are incompatible with the American way of thinking. Americans have been educated to believe that you have to "go to your doctor" for any health advice; that studying and reading about health and practicing sound hygienic and dietetic health principles is the pastime of crackpots and "health nuts." No doubt, this attitude is to a great part responsible for the fact that the average American is so ignorant regarding his own health and the proper means of maintaining it. We are health conscious, yes—but only superficially. We are very confused and ignorant as to what are the correct means, nutritionally and otherwise, to assure optimum health. The lack of reliable expert information on the subject has, perhaps, something to do with this situation. Due to the utterly commercialized nature of the American way of life, most of the chief sources of information, including the government, have some financial and economic interests behind them and thus information often is colored by the influence of these interests.

How to Fast for Lasting Benefits

With this introduction, let me now give a short description of the mechanics of fasting with juices.

First, it is advisable to prepare yourself for fasting with a short cleansing diet. For a day or two before fasting with juice eat nothing but raw fruits and raw vegetables, possibly a few cooked vegetable dishes and yogurt.

On the evening before a fast starts, omit the last meal and take a double enema. Enemas during fasting are taken to help the body eliminate toxins and waste matter from the colon and lower bowels. This is a standard practice in all Swedish biological clinics. An enema is usually taken before retiring. First take about one pint of plain, warmed water, about body temperature, into the bowels and then let it out. Repeat this procedure with a full quart.

The next day—and each following day of the fast—you follow this program:

UPON ARISING:	One single enema, one quart.
8:00 A.M.	Big bowl of vegetable broth.*
11:00 A.M.	Cup of herb tea.*
1:00 P.M.	Glass of freshly pressed fruit juice: orange, apple, grape, pear, etc. Juice should be diluted half-and-half with water.
OR:	Glass of freshly made vegetable juice: carrot juice,* carrot-celery juice,* tomato juice, etc.
4:00 P.M.	Cup of herb tea.
7:00 P.M.	Glass of freshly pressed vegetable juice.
9:00 P.M.	Enema.

Drink plain, warmed water when thirsty.

This is the entire fasting procedure. Again, I would advise, if at all possible, to get your fasting supervised by someone who is quite familiar with the procedures. Under expert supervision such fasting could be undertaken at home up to 30-40 days, if necessary. If you cannot get expert advice, and if you, yourself, are not sufficiently convinced nor well-informed on this therapeutic measure, I would not advise fasting longer than one week or ten days at a time.

How to Break a Fast

Of vital importance is the method of *breaking a fast*. This is the most significant phase of the cycle and the beneficial effects of fasting could be totally undone if a fast is broken incorrectly. The main rules of breaking a fast are: (1) do not overeat; (2) chew extremely well. On the first day, add only one whole apple or other sweet fruit and a little bowl of fresh vegetable salad to the usual juice and broth menu. Next day, add to the above some yogurt and cottage cheese. On the following day increase the portions a little and add some cereal, possibly

* See Chapter 29 for recipe.

some cooked vegetable like baked potato or vegetable soup. Finally, on the fourth day, you can start to eat normally. By "normally" I mean stay on the diet outlined in Chapter 9 of this book. However, always keep in mind the first rule of breaking the fast—do not overeat!

In order to benefit from therapeutic fasting to the greatest possible extent it is important that after the fast a diet of vital, natural foods be maintained. Such a diet will supply the healing forces of the body with all the nutritive elements they need for repair and healing.

It is advisable during fasting to continue with normal activities, but not to do overly strenuous physical or mental work. Daily walks, even long ones, are recommended; also all suitable exercises are very helpful. Baths can be taken, but avoid water which is too cold or too hot. Fresh air is important for the healing processes during fasting. Always sleep with a window open.

Fasting affects many physiological changes in the body. Increased elimination of toxins through urine, skin, and lungs takes place. The body's healing forces will initiate great repair and health-restoring activity in many ways. All these physiological changes may occasionally manifest in certain discomforts, such as headache, coated tongue, foul breath, dizziness. These reactions should, however, give no cause for concern. They are common symptoms of fasting and properly understood should not discourage anybody from continuing with the fast.

Will you feel hungry during your fast? Yes, during the first three days there is a feeling of hunger or a desire for food. But after the third day the hunger usually disappears. In the case of juice fasts, even during the first three days the patient hardly feels any hunger at all.

Above all, the mental attitude during fasting is of vital importance. Avoid negative influences. Do not listen to terrified relatives and "friends" who will warn you that you will pass out at any moment. Nobody ever has died as a result of a few weeks of intentional fasting. But if you do not have complete faith in the fast and are not absolutely convinced of its safety, you should not undertake fasting at all. At least not on your own.

If it makes you feel better, do not call this measure fasting—call it a liquid diet instead. After all, that is exactly what it is.

I know you will be surprised at the results and enjoy the experience. I have fasted myself many times and will never cease to be amazed at the miraculous effects of this the oldest therapeutic method. It was used by Plato and Socrates to "attain mental and physical efficiency." Pythagoras fasted for long periods up to 40 days. Hippocrates, the Father of Medicine, prescribed fasting. And the great physician Paracelsus had said, "Fasting is the greatest remedy."

Chapter 18

What Exercises Are Best
for Arthritis?

First, all exercises should be planned in accordance with the individual needs and capabilities of the patient. No two cases are alike and, consequently, only a general outline of the program can be given here.

As was pointed out before, the body afflicted with arthritis usually suffers from poor circulation, stagnation, and sluggishness. Restoration of the proper circulation is, therefore, essential before the body can effectively accomplish its own healing task. The bloodstream carries fresh oxygen and nutritive elements to all the tissues and organs of the body. It also carries toxic waste materials from the tissues to the eliminative organs where they are expelled from the system. Thus, effective circulation is imperative for successful results in any program of treatment for arthritis.

There are many ways to stimulate circulation, such as

139

massage, alternating hot and cold baths, dry brush massage, etc. But physical exercise in the fresh air is one of the most effective ways to rebuild circulation. For this reason outdoor walking is the most popular form of exercise in all biological clinics.

Of course we should not forget that often a patient is in such a weak condition that he is unable to take any walks. Also, if joints are badly inflamed and painful no exercises should be taken at all—such a patient needs rest more than exercises. But as soon as pain has subsided, immediately a gradually increasing program of exercises should be initiated.

Outside walking is the simplest and most effective way to assist your body's healing and health restoring processes. It will stimulate your glands to secrete more hormones. It will accelerate your metabolism and digestion. It will saturate your blood and all the cells of the body with fresh oxygen. It will assist your eliminative organs in their detoxifying work through the lungs, skin, and intestines. Moreover, a walk in the fresh air, especially in the woods or some other beautiful natural surroundings, will put you in good spirits, stimulate your thinking, and make you feel happy and jubilant all over.

In addition to walking, various other exercises could be used, such as deep-breathing exercises, arm and leg exercises, etc. All this should be adjusted to the condition and ability of the patient. When any particular joint or part of the body is affected it should first be exercised very slowly and, as the movements become freer, the exercises could be gradually accelerated.

To summarize the answer to the question: What exercises are best for arthritis?, I must say that all specific exercises of various joints, limbs, and other parts of the body should be carefully planned in accordance with the needs of each individual case and preferably under expert supervision. However, of far greater importance to the recovery of the patient are various forms of "natural" exercise in fresh air: walking, riding bicycling, swimming, dancing, horse riding, playing games, or any kind of suitable outdoor work, such as gardening. I am a firm believer in natural exercises that give you the benefit of physical exertion without much will effort while simultaneously giving you emotional and spiritual stimulation and enjoyment.

Chapter 19

Are Citrus Fruits Harmful?

In this country, the idea of having some citrus fruit or citrus juice every day is so popularly spread and associated with the concept of a wholesome diet, that even a suggestion of citrus being anything but beneficial is met with skepticism.

Let me state right at the beginning that there is nothing wrong with citrus fruit *per se*. All fruits, including oranges, lemons, and grapefruits, are excellent foods and used with wisdom and in moderation could constitute an important part of every diet.

However, in recent years many nutritionists and medical researchers have questioned the value of citrus in the diet. It was shown in tests that citric acid in citrus fruit can cause tooth damage.[1,2] It has also been shown that citrus juices are linked with peptic ulcers and can unfavorably affect the general

[1] *Journal of Nutrition*, January 10, 1951.
[2] *Journal of the American Dental Association*, May, 1947.

health.[3,4] Some nutritionists and health writers, impressed by the findings of these researchers, have concluded that all citrus fruits should be eliminated from the diet.

It seems to me that the citrus question has been handled rather unscientifically. It is unfair to condemn citrus fruit as such when so many other factors related to its use are not taken into consideration.

First, in tests, which put citrus fruit in a bad light, usually only *citrus juices* are used, not the *whole fruit.*

Second, most citrus fruit in this country has not been given a chance to ripen fully on the trees. They are harvested unripened to assure an early market. Unripe citrus has a much higher content of acids, which can be very harmful, even when the fruit is eaten whole. It is, of course, even more injurious in the form of a concentrated juice.

Third, we should not forget that citrus fruit today is so loaded with toxic chemicals of various kinds—preservatives, artificial colorings, insecticide sprays, waxes, etc.—that some of these are bound to be consumed; this is especially true in regard to commercial juices, where the whole fruit, skin and all, is squeezed in huge, powerful presses.

Then, how many of us do use *fresh* juices anymore? The great majority of Americans drink frozen, reconstituted, or canned fruit juices, not to mention so-called fruit drinks, where there is actually not much of real juice or fruit at all, only artificial colorings and flavorings and various chemicals and preservatives.

Citrus fruits are rich in vitamin C, which is very important for arthritis sufferers, because it is essential for the health and stability of collagen and all connective tissues of the body, as well as for all vital processes of the body and proper functioning of organs and glands. The juice of half a lemon in a glass of warm water, sweetened with one teaspoon of honey, is an

[3] *North Carolina Medical Journal,* November, 1948.
[4] *Oral Surgery, Oral Medicine, and Oral Pathology,* July, 1951.

excellent morning drink for anybody, including persons with arthritis. But it should not be taken every day for prolonged periods. It should be alternated with vegetable broths and herb teas.

Likewise, half a grapefruit once or twice a week, or one whole orange two or three times a week, will do no harm but lots of good. Again it should not be continued endlessly, but alternated with periods when other fruits are used.

The modern, efficient communication and cold storage system makes it possible to buy any kind of fruits and vegetables, anywhere in the United States, any time of the year. This is called progress. But from a nutritional point of view this is a very unfortunate development. This is admittedly great "marketing progress," but it has contributed to the establishment of such unhealthy habits as using certain fruits or, which is even worse, certain fruit juices *every day of the year, year after year.*

All fruit should be eaten "in season." Eat citrus only for a few months during winter when it is harvested. Then switch to the other fruits as they come "in season"—various berries, peaches, cherries, apples, etc. This way you will get fruit always when it is fresh and at the peak of its nutritional value, and your body will be afforded an opportunity to obtain a great variety of nutritive elements. In storage, even cold storage, all produce gradually loses its vitamin content.

The nutritive value of various fruits—vitamins, minerals, enzymes, trace elements, etc.—varies considerably. Also, the habit of eating fruit in season will be a good protective measure for possible damage by an overdosage, as is the case with citric acid in citrus fruits.

In summary, citrus fruits are good for you if you eat them whole and in moderation, not more than two to three in a week. (Lemon is an exception. It can be juiced and used diluted in water in drinks and in salad dressing.) But use citrus only in season and see that it is organically grown without poisonous sprays. In practice, it would mean that you have to buy it only from sources you can trust or from the better health food stores which sell certified, organically grown produce.

If you live in northern parts of the country you can leave citrus fruits out of your diet entirely and replace them with vitamin C-rich apples and other fruits grown in the area.

Chapter 20

What about Cider Vinegar and Honey?

Dr. D. C. Jarvis, M.D., has made apple cider vinegar and honey drink popular in this country. As an exponent of the old Vermont Folk Medicine, he claimed that a simple drink of two teaspoonfuls of apple cider vinegar and two teaspoonfuls of honey in a glass of water at each meal is a cure-all for practically every ill of mankind, including arthritis.[1]

There is considerable doubt in many minds as to the scientific value of this popular remedy.

Now, when I am confronted with an old folk medicine or remedy used for hundreds of years, I investigate it not with a doubt or suspicion, but with a great respect. I reserve my doubts and skepticism for the new toxic chemical drugs which are put on the market daily without much testing or clinical

[1] D. C. Jarvis, M.D., *Arthritis and Folk Medicine*, Holt, Rinehart, and Winston, 1960.

experience as to their true therapeutic value or undesirable side effects.

It seems to me that apple cider vinegar and honey treatment for arthritis may have true merit. People with arthritis are usually in a dilapidated state of health. Their general health is broken down. The functions of the vital organs are weakened and impaired. This is especially true of their digestive and assimilative systems. Most people of middle age and over usually experience diminished secretion of hydrochloric acid in their stomach. This condition leads to poor digestion and consequent inefficient assimilation of nutrients from the foods consumed. This lack of hydrochloric acid in the stomach affects the whole metabolism, especially the mineral metabolism. The disturbed calcium metabolism is but one of the many known contributing causes of arthritis.

Apple cider vinegar and honey drink taken with meals helps to compensate for the insufficient secretion of hydrochloric acid and thus improves digestion of foods. This results in a better assimilation of nutrients and in improved metabolism. Of course, other fruit acids, such as lemon juice, apple juice, or fresh pineapple juice, taken with meals, will accomplish about the same effect.

Honey has many wonderful medicinal properties and is truly one of nature's miracle foods. In biological medicine, honey replaces white sugar whenever a sweetener is needed: in drinks, in foods, etc. Both cider vinegar and honey are beneficial for the digestive tract and exert a favorable influence on constipation, which often accompanies arthritis.

A good use for apple cider vinegar and honey is in making a salad dressing. With cold-pressed vegetable oil and a few natural spices it makes a most delicious and wholesome dressing for fresh vegetable salads. (See Chapter 29 for recipe.)

Warning: ordinary white vinegar is not suitable for these purposes and should never be used. Use only natural apple cider vinegar of health food store quality.

Chapter 21

What about Climate?

There is a general belief that warm climate is good for arthritis and will promote recovery. Arizona has more people afflicted with arthritis than any other state, percentagewise. Thousands of arthritis sufferers come to Arizona, New Mexico, and Southern California in hopes that they will find relief from their agonizing affliction.

Although it is true that hot, dry climate makes arthritics feel more comfortable, it must be emphasized that the change of climate alone is not sufficient to effect a cure and restore health.

I have discussed this question with many prominent doctors in Phoenix, Arizona, who have specialized in treatment of arthritis in that state for a long time. All of them share the opinion that although arthritic patients, who come to Arizona, do feel somewhat better there, they will be quite disappointed if they expect that a change of climate alone will solve their problem.

Dr. C. A. Call, D.C., N.D., has an impressive record of work with arthritic patients. He answered my question thus:

149

"Warm climate and sunbathing are good for people with arthritis, just as they are good for everyone. But they alone cannot cure arthritis. Other treatments, particularly dietetic therapy, must be included."

Dr. R. P. Watterson, M.D., one of the leading medical authorities on treatment of arthritis in Arizona, said to me:

"The warm Arizona climate is of value in treating arthritis, although it is not a decisive factor in effecting a cure. People are outdoors more here in Arizona; they get more fresh, clean air, more ultraviolet rays; they are engaged in more outdoor sports and exercises and perspire more; even the pollen count is less here. All these are beneficial factors. But the change to a hot climate alone will not accomplish a cure. In my experience, arthritis is the end result of a systemic disturbance—a biochemical suffocation and a metabolic impairment. It can be successfully treated only if the underlying nutritional abuses are corrected and a proper biochemical balance is restored."

Then, it should not be forgotten that any kind of a change which takes the patient away from the monotony of the set routine of his daily living, is good for him—emotionally and psychologically. Also, people living in Southern California and Arizona have a better supply of fresh, local fruits and vegetables the year round. They can eat a better and more nutritious than average diet. All these factors contribute to a patient's recovery.

We should never forget that to enable the healing power of the body to function more efficiently and accomplish a cure, we must support it by establishing and maintaining the most favorable environment and conditions for such healing functions to take place. All the positive factors, such as diet, baths, fasting, vitamin and mineral supplements, etc., are beneficial and welcomed. The warm, dry climate, conducive to vigorous outdoor life and exposure to sunlight and fresh air, is just *one* of these positive factors.

Chapter 22

Should Arthritis Sufferers Adhere to a High-Protein Diet?

Americans have been so brainwashed with the "high-protein" idea that it makes me feel like a heretic of sorts to try to discredit this high-protein myth.

Everybody from a schoolchild to grandma "knows" that a *high-protein, low-carbohydrate* diet is best for your health. You read this in the medical, syndicated columns of your daily newspaper; you hear this on TV and radio commercials; you read about it in the popular health magazines and in books on nutrition by the "experts." We all have been fed this propaganda and been geared for the high-protein cult for decades—from all possible directions, even from roadside billboards and "beef for health" stickers on automobile bumpers! We are advised by "authorities" to eat *lots* of meat, eggs, fish, and milk and to get as much protein as possible. In fact, many nutritionists will tell you that you can never get too much protein. And in our kindly American way we feel sorry for all the poor people

151

in "underdeveloped" countries who "don't get enough protein."

How did this false myth originate? I don't really know. Maybe meat-packing industries have some part to play in it. Or perhaps the scientific fact that our bodies are made up mostly of proteins is responsible for it. Whatever the reason, our present nutritional and medical, as well as general public thinking is in complete accord concerning the necessity of a high-protein diet for good health.

The Facts about Protein Diet

At the risk of disappointing many steak lovers, I must state that *there is no scientific truth* in the high-protein-for-health theory. If you are really concerned with your health and long life, you must unlearn everything you have learned previously concerning proteins.

It is true that our bodies are built mostly of proteins. Twenty per cent, and more in some vital organs, of a cell's composition is made up of protein. Since our body is renewing and repairing its cells constantly, we need lots of protein in our diet to supply needed nutrients for these repairs and for the building of new cells.

But how much is "lots"? Seventy, 100, or 150 grams a day, as advocated by many American "experts"? Due to the frame of this work we cannot, unfortunately, go into great detail in presenting this most interesting subject. Suffice here to say that the majority of responsible nutritionists in various parts of the world agree that our present beliefs on the protein question are outdated and that the actual need for protein in the human diet is far below that which has long been considered necessary. The famous nutritionists Dr. Ragnar Berg, Dr. R. Chittenden, Dr. M. Hindhede, Dr. M. Hegsted, Dr. William C. Rose, and others are reported to have shown in extensive experiments that our actual need for protein is somewhere around 30 grams a day, or even less. Many leading contemporary scientists and nutritionists in Europe, such as Dr. Ralph Bircher, Dr. Otto Buchinger, Jr., Dr. H. Karström, Prof. H. A. Schweigart, Dr. Karl-Otto Aly, and many others are in full agreement with the findings of Drs. Berg, Chittenden, Rose, et al., and are recommending a *low-protein diet* as the diet most conducive to good health.

Empirical experience and observation proves the correctness of the above fact. The healthiest people in the world—the famous Hunza people in India, the semitic tribes of Yemen, Bulgarians and Russians, certain tribes of Central America and Africa—which are known for their good health, long life, and resistance to disease, all live on a low animal protein, high natural carbohydrate diet. Even in the United States, some religious groups, like the Seventh-Day Adventists and Mormons, who advocate a low animal protein diet, have 50 to 70 per cent *lower death rates* than those of average Americans; this is shown by statistics. They also are reported to have a much *lower incidence* of cancer, tuberculosis, coronary diseases, blood and kidney diseases, and diseases of the digestive and respiratory organs.[1,2]

Protein's Role in Metabolism

The chemical composition of proteins is well known but their biological properties and their full role in the metabolic processes is not too well understood, and perhaps never will be. We know that proteins in the body are in the so-called *dynamic* state. This means they are constantly being changed from one state to another, being decomposed and resynthesized from the blood plasma amino acids. This phenomenon, perhaps, may help to solve the protein cult mystery. It is claimed that we need a new protein supply, "lots of it," *every day*. The fact is,

[1] John A. Widtsoe and Leah D. Widtsoe, *The Word of Wisdom,* Deseret Books, 1950.
[2] Dr. Frank R. Lemon and Dr. Richard T. Walden, *Journal of the American Medical Association,* October, 1966.

however, that our body can exist without *any* food, and consequently without *any proteins,* for weeks and months, as for instance in the case of complete therapeutic fasting. And not only without harm but with evident health benefits! The reason for this is that our body has a way of decomposing and re-synthesizing proteins and reusing them again where they are needed. Protein stored in the liver is converted to plasma proteins, which then supply the cells with needed amino acids.

The greatest fault of the high-protein diet is that all protein in excess of the actual need is burned up as energy or stored in the body as fat. Also, the digestion of animal protein causes building of certain toxins. Nitrogen is transformed to uric acid which exerts an added stress on kidneys and the liver.[3] It also causes intestinal poisoning through putrefaction. In the case of weakened kidneys and impairment in the functioning of other eliminative organs, toxic wastes are deposited in the tissues and may cause autointoxication and sluggishness—the factors usually associated with development of arthritis. Particularly for arthritis sufferers it is important to adopt a *low animal protein diet.* Dr. D. C. Jarvis, M.D., in his book on arthritis stresses this point and advocates a diet high in natural carbo-hydrates and low in animal proteins, especially meat.[4]

Although the majority of medical physicians, encouraged by the official support of AMA and the National Arthritis Foundation, stubbornly persist in their belief that nutrition has nothing to do with the cause or cure of arthritis, there is an encouragingly growing number of more progressive physi-cians who are beginning to realize the vital role nutrition plays in the development and management of this crippling disease. Particularly, the currently fashionable high-protein cult is under suspicion as a possible culprit in many diseases, including arthritis. At the annual meeting of the New York Rheumatism

[3] Dr. Irving Fisher and Dr. Eugene Lyman Fisk, *How to Live.*
[4] D. C. Jarvis, M.D., *Arthritis and Folk Medicine,* Holt, Rinehart, and Winston, 1960

Foundation, Dr. Donald A. Gerber, assistant professor of medicine at New York University, stated that development of rheumatoid arthritis could be caused by a defect in body chemistry which interferes with the metabolism of protein. He then suggested that a low-protein diet may provide the answer to sufferers of this painful affliction.[5]

In the biological program of treatments for arthritis, meat and fish are always excluded completely. The only animal proteins used are milk and cheese. The importance of the vegetable protein foods, such as beans, nuts, grains, and especially soybeans, is emphasized.

One fact overlooked by proponents of the high animal protein diet is that, according to experiments by many prominent scientists (Schweigart, Rose, and others), some *vegetable proteins* are of as good or better biological value than *animal proteins*. The Journal of the American Medical Association reported that protein derived in a proportion of up to two thirds from plant origin is entirely adequate in quality to meet all protein needs required for normal growth and sustenance of health.[6] Vegetable proteins—grains, beans, seeds, nuts, green plants, potatoes, etc.—consumed in variety and fortified with milk and cheese, will supply you with all the essential amino acids, or complete proteins, needed for perfect health.

TO SUMMARIZE, you need to be sure that good proteins are included in your diet. Proteins are essential to insure proper functioning of all your vital organs. But you must see that your diet does not contain too much animal protein. A high animal protein diet may cause such disturbances as overacidity, internal putrefaction, constipation, uric acid in blood and tissues, high blood pressure, high blood cholesterol level, obesity, etc. and be a predisposing factor in development of arthritis.

[5] *New York Times*, April 7, 1965.
[6] "Nutritional Contributions of Wheat," *the Journal of AMA*, November 29, 1948.

Chapter 23

Are Vitamin and Mineral
Supplements Necessary?

There can be no doubt that the state and quality of your nutrition is directly related to the state and quality of your health. I don't think there is any disagreement among the majority of nutritionists and health authorities on the importance of good, well-balanced, vitamin- and mineral-rich nutrition for the optimum of health and vitality. Vital nutrition is the major determining factor for the state of your health. The vitamins and minerals you eat—or don't eat—can make a colossal difference in the way you look and feel. Nutritional deficiencies are generally considered to be contributing factors in so-called degenerative diseases, including arthritis.

So far so good, and everybody is in full accord: vital nutrition —vitamins, minerals, complete proteins, carbohydrates, essential fatty acids, trace elements, enzymes, etc.—is essential both for the maintenance of good health and the prevention of disease. The discord starts when we try to determine how we can obtain all these nesessary nutrients and guard ourselves against nutritional deficiencies.

The"official" thinking, represented by many governmental health organizations and conservative food researchers, is that you can get your vitamins "with knife and fork." That is, if you eat a "well-balanced diet" you will be well nourished. They claim that vitamin and mineral supplements are a waste of money and absolutely unnecessary, except in cases determined by your doctor and prescribed by him. The vociferous champion of the food processing industry, Dr. Frederick Stare, Harvard University nutritionist, claims that we are the best-fed nation in the world, that ordinary foods available at any grocery store, including white bread, sugar, and processed and canned foods, will produce "just as good nutritional health as any and all health foods." Moreover, he maintains that the only ones who benefit from vitamins and food supplements are the vitamin and food supplement manufacturers and retailers.

The second point of view, held by many of the world's most prominent nutritionists, biochemists, and progressive medical researchers is that while under ideal conditions—100 per cent natural, poison-free foods and environment—we should not need any food supplements at all, but under present conditions, especially in the United States, food supplements are imperative if health and vitality are to be maintained.

Can you get your vitamins with a knife and fork, as many authorities today advise you? And isn't this the most natural and sound way to assure proper nutrition?

Indeed it is! In principle, a well-chosen and well-balanced diet of nutritionally sound, unprocessed, natural, unadulterated foods (grown in undepleted, fertile soils without poisonous sprays) will give you all the vitamins, minerals, proteins, enzymes, and trace elements you need without any addition or food supplements. A hundred or even 50 years ago such advice would have been both sound and workable. Your grandparents drank pure, unpolluted water, breathed clear air without carbon monoxide and other pollutants, and ate wholesome foods which were organically grown on their own farm. They ate fresh fruits and vegetables from their own garden; cereals grown in a well-manured field; meat, eggs, and dairy products from their own healthy farm animals. Processed and refined foods were all but unknown. Candies, commercially produced soft drinks, and canned foods were luxuries which only the rich could afford. Whatever unhealthy foods or living habits they had were well counteracted and worked off by vigorous physical activity outdoors which farm life demanded of them.

The fruits and vegetables they ate had no residues of poisonous sprays and waxes, and they contained more vitamins than artificially grown produce of today. The eggs your grandparents ate were fertile eggs, produced by hens eating worms, bugs, grass, etc. in addition to the natural grains. Such eggs had much higher vitamin, mineral, and lecithin content than today's eggs, produced in egg factories by chicks which never see the sunlight and eat chemicalized mash. The wheat from which your grandparents' bread was made contained a minimum of 18 plus per cent protein, often as high as 24 per cent. Your "enriched bread" is made from wheat grown on depleted soils with chemical fertilizers, which has reduced its protein content to an average below 10 per cent![1] Not to mention the fact that over 40 vital nutritional elements have been removed from it, including vitamin E, and then "enriched" with four synthetic, biologically inferior drugs! Meat and dairy products today are packed with preservatives, DDT, hormones, and other chemicals and drugs which were unknown 100 years ago.

It is a well-known fact that due to vitamin, protein, and enzyme-destroying practices of the food producing and food

[1] Dr. W. F. Chappelle, D.D.S., *Quality Foods for Health*, Lee Foundation for Nutritional Research.

processing industries our modern-day foods are nutritionally *not the same* as the natural foods which haven't been over-processed or refined.

As you can see, what was considered to be a sound and ideal practice yesterday, cannot be realized today; at least not in this overcivilized country. What was yesterday's law is today's folly. Many Americans today are attempting to get their vitamins with a knife and fork, but they still fall short of optimum nutritional standards. The reason for this, of course, is that virtually all the foods you buy at your supermarket today are nutritionally inferior one way or the other. So it doesn't matter how well you balance your meals, if you are a meat-eater, vegetarian, or health faddist, you still run a chance of malnutrition, because food processors and manufacturers have removed or destroyed many of the vital nutrients from the food you buy.

Perhaps it would be possible today to obtain all your vitamins and other nutritive elements with knife and fork if you were a very well-informed and enlightened nutritionist with a scientific medical and biochemical background. But for the average housewife it is quite impossible to orient herself among the glittering aisles of brightly colored plastic wraps and gaudy labels of modern supermarkets and make an intelligent choice of foods, nutritionally speaking.

Therefore, most people either can't or don't take the time and effort to eat a nutritionally balanced diet. They eat the "average American diet" loaded with refined carbohydrates, soft drinks, crackers, white bread, ice cream, cakes and pies, canned and frozen foods, processed sugared cereals, coffee and toast, TV dinners, and such. This atrocious diet of devitalized foods is the major reason why our health standards are among the lowest in the world, as health statistics show. Our mortality rate is steadily increasing and is higher than the rates in many so-called underdeveloped countries. To be exact, 88 nations of the world have a lower death rate than we have.[2] The physical and mental health of our children is far below the record of European children, as was shown in recent comparable tests. A ten year study of American youngsters between the ages of 13 and 20, in which 2,536 boys and girls participated, has shown that almost half of them suffered from "nutritional nerves," (which usually indicate lack of vitamin B-complex), insufficient protein in their diets, and serious- shortages of vitamins A, B, and C.[3] Several surveys indicate that only about one-half of the school children in America get enough vitamin C in their diet. It is a well-established medical fact that an alarming percentage of our population suffers from nutritional deficiencies, notably of calcium and vitamin C.

Dr. Robert S Coodhart, president of the National Vitamin Foundation, at a recent (October, 1966) conference of the Foundation, attended by 30 of the nation's leading nutrition scientists, said: "We know that such things as the determination of vitamin levels in tissue fluids, the taking of diet histories, and physical examinations for external signs of nutrient deficiencies are not sufficient, by themselves or in combination, to permit us to arrive at valid conclusions about the incidence and importance to health of degree of malnutrition, short of gross undernutrition or gross overnutrition." Subclinical malnutrition and vitamin deficiencies are more common in the United States than is generally known. The U. S. Department of Agriculture findings indicate that in 48 per cent of U. S. households diets do not fully meet "normal" allowances for essential vitamins and other nutrients!

These bad nutritional patterns of empty calories should be changed and the American people should be educated in better eating habits. But this cannot be done overnight. People will

[2] "Population and Vital Statistics Report," *United Nations*, Vol. XVIII, No. 2, April 1, 1966.
[3] "Starved Adolescents," *Newsweek*, Mar. 4, 1953.

continue to buy and eat worthless foods. Skillful, never-ending advertising by the powerful commercial interests of the food processing industry will see to that.

Here's where the food supplements come in. The prime purpose of food supplements is to fill in nutritional gaps left by faulty eating habits.

Food supplements return to your diet what food processors have removed or destroyed. Many vital nutritional elements, particularly enzymes and vitamins, are completely destroyed by modern food processing and refining methods.

It is a medically well-known fact that even minor deficiencies of one or more of the vital nutritive factors will result in disturbed chemistry in the system, lowered resistance to infections, and can cause various diseases.

Thus, food supplements are a nutritional insurance against disease. Well-chosen food supplements are an easy, practical, and inexpensive way to improve your deficient diet and assure optimum health for you and your family.

Another important reason for taking food supplements is that they will protect you from the harmful effects of poisonous additives and residues in your food, water, and air. Many vitamins possess antipoison properties, especially vitamin C. Vitamins C, B, and E will help to protect you against many insecticide residues, which you just can't avoid. Bone meal will protect you from harmful effects of Strontium 90, which none of us can avoid getting into our systems these days. The toxic effects of smoking and drinking (both nicotine and alcohol are known vitamin antagonists) are modified by heavy doses of vitamins C and B. Desiccated liver tablets, wheat germ, and wheat germ oil will protect you and your heart from stress and increase your endurance. In this poisoned world of ours, where lethal poisons are lurking in all directions—in air, water, food, clothing, etc.—food supplements are virtually your only available protection against their harmful effects.

If the above is true for the average person, it is doubly true for one who is afflicted with arthritis. As I have shown before, *faulty eating habits and nutritional deficiencies are the major environmental factors leading to an onset of arthritis.* Therefore, the first step in a successful program of treatments should be a complete overhaul of nutritional habits. An improved diet of vital foods as outlined in this book, fortified with well-chosen food supplements, will supply your body with all the vitamins, proteins, minerals, enzymes, and trace elements needed for its healing and health-restoring processes.

Chapter 24

Which Food Supplements Should I Take?

Nutrition is a relatively new science, barely 30 years old. It has already made impressive gains in knowledge. But we have only scratched the surface. In coming years nutritionists will discover and identify many new vitamins and other nutritional factors which will play an important role in your health.

Therefore, one who does not suffer from any specific disease or deficiency but who is interested in food supplements for prophylactic or preventive reasons—that is for health protection —should not take any vitamins, minerals, or other isolated factors. But he should use natural food supplements, such as brewer's yeast, kelp, bone meal, rose hips, cold-pressed vegetable oils, cod liver oil, wheat germ oil, etc. These are all natural, unrefined *foods*, rather than isolated vitamins or minerals. When you take them you will be benefiting not only from all the known vitamins and other nutritional factors, but also from all the unknown, as yet undiscovered, factors. Moreover, in such natural food supplements all the vital factors are present in their naturally balanced combination. This is important for two reasons. First, this will assure their full biological activity and maximum assimilation. Second, it will prevent overdosage which, as in the cases of vitamins D, A, and certain vitamins of the B-complex, could be quite dangerous.

The above remarks are made in reference to relatively healthy people. In the case of disease, however, the use of isolated vitamins and other nutritional factors could be not only justified but, in many cases, absolutely essential.

Vitamins

In arthritis, most clinics in Sweden use certain vitamins and mineral preparations in addition to the other dietetic measures.

Impaired adrenal function is one of the major characteristics of arthritis. It has been shown that prolonged deficiencies of vitamin C and two B vitamins, pantothenic acid and B2, can severely damage the adrenals and result in decreased cortisone production. Vitamin C increases the production and the utilization of cortisone.[1]

Therefore, the majority of biologically oriented doctors advise heavy doses of vitamin C in treatment of arthritis. This should be a natural vitamin C, made from rose hips, acerola berries, green peppers, or other natural sources. Arthritis sufferers are advised to take up to 1,500 milligrams of vitamin C each day. Natural vitamin C, in addition to ascorbic acid, contains bioflavonoids—citrin, hesperidin, rutin—which always accompany vitamin C in its natural state, and, when consumed together, make ascorbic acid biologically more effective and potent than a synthetic, pure ascorbic acid.

Another vitamin used in arthritis is vitamin B-12. Dr. Lars-Erik Essén of Vita Nova has used it with good results.

[1] *Nutritional Review,* 13, 1955 and 15, 1957

Vitamin E is also considered very useful in the treatment of arthritis. It is suggested by some researchers that the scar tissue, which forms around the joints in arthritis, could develop as a result of vitamin E deficiency. Reported recommended dosage is 300-600 I.U. a day.[2]

Pantothenic acid is another vitamin which plays an important role in the development of arthritis. Studies have shown that people with arthritis have extremely low levels of many vitamins in their blood, particularly vitamin C and pantothenic acid.[3] Dr. R. J. Williams has suggested that persons with arthritis may have unusually high requirements for pantothenic acid.[4] It might be wise to supplement the diet of an arthritis sufferer with pantothenic acid. Doses of 100 to 500 milligrams a day have been reported during shorter periods of treatment, reduced later to 100 milligrams a day.

Minerals

Minerals are also considered extremely important in the treatment of arthritis. Disturbance in the body's mineral metabolism is usually indicated in arthritis. Therefore, the restoration of proper mineral balance in the tissues is imperative for effective and fast recovery.

Various mineral supplements are used by different practitioners. For the United States, the mineral supplements most useful and easily available would be kelp and bone meal. Recommended doses are about five kelp and five bone meal tablets each day. Both also could be obtained in powder form and taken in a dosage of about one teaspoon of each a day. Kelp is especially beneficial for arthritis sufferers. It could be used as a salt replacement in the seasoning of salads and other foods.

[2] Dr. H. Selye, *Calciphylaxis*, University of Chicago Press, 1962.
[3] L. Eising, *J. Bone Joint Surgery*, 1963.
[4] R. J. Williams, *Biochemical Individuality*, Wiley, New York, 1956.

In Japan, where kelp (seaweed) is used extensively as an important part of the daily diet, arthritis is virtually nonexistent.

Other Supplements

The following food supplements, in addition to the ones mentioned above, are used and recommended by most biologically oriented practitioners:

Brewer's yeast (or food yeast) about 3 tbsp. a day.

Note: never use yeast intended for baking!

Cod liver oil, plain, not fortified—1 tsp. a day.

Raw wheat germ—3 to 5 tbsp. a day.

Wheat germ oil—1 tbsp. a day.

Lecithin (granules or liquid)—1 tbsp. a day.

Whey, tablets or powder (for better intestinal hygiene).

In addition, such natural foods as honey, soybeans, sunflower seeds, sesame seeds, raw nuts, yogurt, black molasses, and cold-pressed vegetable oils should be used liberally to make a diet well balanced and nutritious.

Parenthetically, for best effect and full biological value, all vitamins and minerals and other food supplements should always be taken *with meals*. Because many vitamins are water soluble, and taken in large doses could be readily lost in urine, it is advisable that the daily dose should be evenly divided between three meals, rather than everything taken with one single meal.

Chapter 25

What Role Does Constipation Play in Arthritis?

Constipation is one of the most common ailments of civilized man. It does not exist among primitive people. It is a result of sedentary life in combination with denatured, refined, and devitalized foods—conditions for which our body was not made.

It is a common observation that many people afflicted with arthritis have a long record of chronic constipation preceding the onset of the disease.

Constipation is the root of many evils. It causes great discomfort and can be a contributing or major cause of a great many diseases. It may lead to such disorders as hemorrhoids, varicose veins, hernia, upset digestion, nervous irritability, skin eruptions, eczema, muddy complexion, and headaches. "Bad breath"—a national disgrace on which mouthwash manufacturers are now making millions of dollars—is more often than not a direct result of constipation. (Needless to say, no mouth-wash can correct bad breath caused by constipation, since foul odor comes from the stomach and the lungs, not from the mouth!)

But constipation can also lead to many more serious diseases, such as impaired function of liver, gall bladder, kidneys, and other vital organs, and can be one of the major contributing causes of arthritis.

Your intestines house billions of different bacteria which help your digestive system break down the food you eat and thus aid their housing organism in its metabolic processes. Some of these are what we call "friendly bacteria," some are "unfriendly" or putrefactive bacteria. When the diet is un-balanced, as in the case of too much refined and overcooked carbohydrates and too much animal protein, the balance of the intestinal flora is disturbed, harmful bacteria take over, and the result is sluggish bowels, gas, putrefaction, and con-stipation. Toxins (poisons) created by bacterial metabolism and putrefaction remain in the intestines and, as a result of prolonged constipation, are absorbed by the bloodstream, poisoning the whole organism. Chronic constipation will even-tually weaken the muscles of the large intestine so that they will not be able to function properly and expel waste matter from the colon. Chronically constipated and sluggish intestines lead to chronic autointoxication or self-poisoning.

As was pointed out in Chapter 6, the impaired elimination of metabolic wastes and toxins from the system, and resultant autointoxication, is one of the most prominent syndromes or characteristics of arthritis. Therefore, those afflicted with ar-thritis should make a special effort to overcome constipation—this largely ignored and neglected but very dangerous ailment. Even if you do not suffer from arthritis as yet, but are badly constipated, make sure you correct this trouble before it leads to more serious complications.

How Do You Know When You Are Constipated?

Most people will say that they are all right, their bowels move once a day. Many are satisfied when they evacuate only once every two or three days. If your bowels move only once in two or three days you are *badly* constipated, even if you don't feel pain or discomfort at present. Such delayed evacuation will eventually, more likely than not, lead to serious illnesses. But even if your bowels move once every day, intestinal sluggishness is definitely indicated.

People living under natural, primitive conditions move their bowels after each meal. Most animals do the same. Healthy infants follow the same pattern. Adults, too, should do likewise. They should at least evacuate twice a day, morning and evening.

Constipation can be corrected only by adopting a sound, commonsense program of natural foods, proper eating habits, plenty of exercise, plenty of liquids, and establishing a habit of regular routine. Laxatives will never solve this colossal health problem. They only weaken the natural functions of the intestines and ultimately cause more harm than good.

The sufferers of arthritis who avail themselves of biological treatments as outlined in this book, will have their constipation problems automatically solved. Fasting, enemas, and "eliminative diets" of raw foods will effectively rebuild and restore the normal function of the intestinal organs and bring about good elimination.

A Program to Conquer Constipation

Here is a seven-point, do-it-yourself program to solve your constipation problem forever—the natural way.

1. Eat plenty of raw fruits and vegetables. Eat several pieces of any available raw fruit and a big bowl of fresh green vegetable salad every day. Chew all your foods well.

2. Avoid constipating foods: meat, white bread, processed cereals, refined carbohydrates (such as sugar, cakes, candies, ice cream, and such).

3. Eat soaked prunes (six to ten) with your breakfast. A bowl of yogurt with half a dozen prunes, two tablespoons of wheat germ, and one tablespoon of bran is a royal dish to start your day with. Do not cook prunes, just wash them well, put them in a cup of warm water and soak them overnight. Important: be sure to drink the water in which the prunes were soaked!

4. Supplement your diet with brewer's yeast, whey powder, honey, and yogurt—all natural laxatives.

5. Exercise! Walk, swim, ride, dance, play golf—anything at all, but exercise! Lack of sufficient exercise—physical inactivity—is one of the main causes of constipation. Plain walking is one of the best forms of exercise. Start with an hour's walking a day!

6. Consume plenty of liquids: water, juice (unsweetened only), broth, soups—six to eight glasses a day.

7. Never suppress nature's call! Try immediately upon arising and again before retiring to establish a habit of bowel movements. Be careful not to overstrain—just relax and wait, if needed up to ten to 15 minutes. This will eventually result in a well-established routine.

If you follow this seven-point program conscientiously, you can safely throw away all your laxatives. You will never need them again, unless you are already a pathological case with a completely atrophied and degenerated eliminative system. Then you will need a prolonged program of fasting, enemas, special diets, exercises, and other biological treatments under the careful supervision of an understanding practitioner. But even the most obstinate types of constipation can be overcome if proper biological treatments, fortified with patience and steadfastness, are applied.

Chapter 26

Can Injuries and Physical Stress Cause Arthritis?

Patients afflicted with arthritis are usually in a condition of exhaustion and chronic fatigue. Studies also reveal that most persons with arthritis have been under severe stress for prolonged periods before onset of the disease.

In order to give an intelligent answer to the question: "Can injuries and stress cause arthritis?", we must first agree on the definition of the word "stress."

In a way, all diseases are caused by stress. That is, if we give the word "stress" a meaning which modern medical thinking has given to it in recent years. According to the greatest authority on stress, famous Dr. Hans Selye, of the University of Montreal, Canada, stress could be defined as anything that harms or damages the body.[1] Stress is not only what the general public means when it talks about the "stresses of

[1] Dr. Hans Selye, *The Stress of Life*, McGraw-Hill, New York, 1956.

modern living." Included also are such things as bacterial and viral infections, insufficient or unbalanced diet, inadequate sleep, lack of exercise, and nutritional deficiencies. Of course, anxiety, mental exhaustion, and constant worries and fears are more commonly understood forms of stress. But such things as x-ray, most drugs, constipation, polluted air, toxic residues in foods, fever, tissue damage (by sprain, blows, or cuts), pain, poor appetite. bad digestion, sweating, vomiting, etc. are all forms of stress

Now, when man is in perfect health, enjoys adequate nutrition, has a strong, healthy body and mind, possesses a clean bloodstream, and has all the vital organs and glands in tip-top working condition—most, if not all, injuries and stresses can be easily overcome, needed repairs can be made quickly, and no serious deleterious aftereffects are left. In other words, if you are healthy you don't get sick! But how many of us can qualify for the above description of perfect health?

Injuries and undue physical strains to the joints or other parts of the body can contribute to the development of arthritis if the body is already in a debilitated state, suffers from serious nutritional deficiencies, and/or is overloaded with accumulated toxins. In such a case, the damaged joints or muscle can become the focal point of the disease.

Thus, injuries and stresses, *per se*, do not cause arthritis, but they may contribute to its development when the body's resistance is lowered.

Dr. Hans Selye refers to arthritis as one of the "stress diseases." Adrenal exhaustion from prolonged stress is one of the major causes leading to the development of arthritis. The pituitary and/or adrenal glands, due to prolonged stress and consequent impaired metabolism, are no longer able to function normally and produce cortisone, desoxycortisone, aldosterone, and other hormones. Severe hormonal imbalance will be the result which leads to a further metabolic derangement and severely lowered resistance to further stress from infections, drugs, toxic substances in foods, etc. This is why patients receiving cortisone often have an immediate feeling of well-being—the deficient hormone helps to restore their impaired metabolism. But, of course, as was shown in Chapter 7, the damage this hormone in a synthetic form can cause far outweighs the good it accomplishes.

To make sure that injuries and stresses do not cause permanent damage and lead to the development of serious chronic conditions, such as arthritis, you must see that your general health condition and resistance to disease is always at the optimal level.

"Meeting the demands of stress," as famed nutritionist Adele Davis calls it, should be your first consideration. This could be best done by adopting a new way of life as outlined in this book. The well-balanced diet, which will supply the pituitary and adrenal glands with all the nutrients necessary for adequate hormone production, is an absolute necessity. A diet rich in unprocessed fresh vegetables, fruits, grain, seeds, milk, and milk products will supply your glands with all the needed nutritional elements and keep your body well prepared to meet the "demands of stress."

Let me remind you again that vitamin C is known as an antistress vitamin. Vitamin C stimulates the adrenal glands and increases the production of cortisone.[2] Be sure that you get ample amounts of this vitamin, perhaps the most important one of all. Take up to 1,000-1,500 milligrams a day or even more when under an unusual stress or subject to injuries. Fresh and/or desiccated liver, brewer's yeast, wheat germ, and wheat germ oil are other foods with antistress factors. They are rich in vitamin B-complex, including pantothenic acid, which is known to be an important antistress vitamin, especially in correcting the condition of adrenal exhaustion. Adele Davis recommends supplementing the diet with 400-500 milligrams

[2] B. H. Ershoff, *Nut. Rev.*, 13, 1955.

of pantothenic acid daily, taken 100 mg. at a time, with three to four hour intervals, in times of stress.[3]

Of course, many other vitamins and minerals could be considered as vital antistress factors, especially vitamins E, D, and A. Be sure that your diet is well supplied with all the necessary nutritional elements to keep you well prepared for the "stresses of life."

[3] Adele Davis, *Let's Get Well,* Harcourt, Brace & World, Inc., 1965.

Chapter 27

Is It Possible for an American to Obtain Treatments in European Biological Clinics?

All the clinics which I visited are privately owned and will accept patients from anywhere. I have specifically asked this question and in every case received an affirmative answer.

Of course, the cost of travel to Europe should be considered. On the other hand, the charges in these clinics are usually very low, compared with the fees in American hospitals.

First, here are the names and addresses of Swedish biological clinics which are described in this book:

1. Brandals Hälsohem, Alma Nissen, Pershagen, Sweden.
2. Vita Nova, Dr. Lars-Erik Essén, Mölle, Sweden.
3. Björkagården Hälsohem, Ingrid Öye-Carlson, Djurås, Sweden.

4. Kurhemmet, Dr. Jern Hamberg, Alfta, Sweden.
5. Kiholms Hälsohem, Harry Andersson, Södertälje, Sweden.

Below are some of the most well-known clinics and spas on the European continent which specialize in biological methods of treatment.

1. Privat-Klinik Bircher-Benner, Keltenstr. 48—CH 8044, Zürich, Switzerland.
2. Ringberg-Klinik, Dr. Josef Issels, 8183 Rottach-Egern/Tegernsee, West Germany. (This is the most outstanding clinic in the world for biological cancer therapy.)
3. Klinik Prof. Werner Zabel, 824 Berchtesgaden/Bayern, West Germany.
4. Kurheim, Dr. Trumpp, 8959 Hopfen am See, Switzerland.
5. Diätkurheim "Winter," 7744 Königsfeld-Burgberg, Switzerland.
6. Fasten Sanatorium, Dr. Otto Buchinger (Sen.) Überlingen am Bodensee, West Germany.
7. Fasten-Sanatorium am Bombey, Dr. Otto Buchinger, Jr., Bad Pyrmont (Hannover), West Germany.
8. Abteilung für Naturheilverfahren, Allgemeines Krankenhause, Dr. Fritz Oelze, Hamburg-Ochsenzoll, West Germany.
9. Kurheim, Dr. Ernst Meyer-Camberg, 8124 Seeshaupt am Starnberger See, West Germany.
10. Weserbergland-Klinik, Prof. Dr. Lampert, Hoxter/Weser, West Germany.
11. Paracelsus-haus, Dr. W. Bühler, 7261 Unterlengenhardt, Schwartzwald, West Germany.
12. Biologisches Sanatorium "Haus der Gesundheit," Dr. E. v. Weckbecker, 8788 Brückenau/Bayern, West Germany.

Of the above I especially recommend Privat-Klinik Bircher-Benner, in Zürich and Fasten-Sanatorium am Bombey of Dr. Otto Buchinger, Jr., in Bad Pyrmont. They are both huge clinics each with a large staff of doctors and extensive up-to-date facilities. Klinik Prof. Zabel is also recommended.

Of course, you may write to any of the Swedish clinics which I described in this book. Keep in mind that many clinics are always filled up and it will be necessary to make an early reservation. The clinics will be happy to answer any inquiries concerning the fees, reservations, treatments, etc.

Parenthetically, biological clinics do not guarantee a cure for arthritis or any other disease. No other clinic, hospital, or doctor can honestly do so. This book is based on the actual case histories of men and women who were cured of arthritis or were helped to better their condition through the application of biological methods, as they are practiced by Swedish practitioners. It should not be misconstrued to mean, imply, or indicate that the therapies described in this book will cure all types and all cases of arthritis, as no such claims are made. The human body is a very complex mechanism and every individual reacts differently to any specific treatment. What is meat for one, could be poison for another. Every condition is unique and it is impossible to foresee its exact development. Although the large majority of all cases treated in biological clinics do recover from arthritis, there are cases where destructive pathological changes are so severe and the body's own healing mechanism so weakened that complete correction of the disease is not possible. But even in very advanced and seemingly hopeless cases biological treatments usually arrest further development of the disease. My advice is that sufferers of arthritis should not attempt to treat themselves by the methods described in this book. They should consult a physician who understands the principles of biological medicine and undertake a program of treatment under his expert supervision.

Perhaps this will be an appropriate place to make the following statement:

"I do not have any financial or economic interest in any of

the clinics recommended above, and, needless to say, am not receiving any monetary or other remuneration for recommending them to my readers. I am doing this for one reason only— the same reason which motivated writing this book—to help the millions of arthritis sufferers in any way I can.

"Likewise, I do not own any health food store, nor do I have financial interests in any such store. Also, I am not connected with any vitamin or food supplement manufacturing or retailing industry, in case you have received such an impression after reading my repeated recommendation for food supplements and health food stores."

Chapter 28

How to Find a Biologically Oriented Doctor in the United States

The term biological medicine, as used in this book, is a relatively new expression. Although it is used quite often in Europe, popularly and officially in scientific publications, the average American layman as well as the average physician are not too familiar with it.

The *concept of biological medicine,* on the other hand, is not new at all. It goes back as far as the very early history of the art of healing. It encompasses all the naturopathic, drugless therapies which were practiced for thousands of years, even before Hippocrates. During various periods of medical history and in different parts of the world these methods of healing were and are called by different names. In the United States, the school of healing nearest to the concept of biological medicine, would probably be called naturopathy, nature-cure method, natural hygiene, or drugless medicine. There are numerous naturopathic physicians, chiropractors, and drugless osteopathic physicians in this country who use in their practice methods of treatment very similar to those outlined in this book. Naturopathic physicians particularly would be very sympathetic towards biological therapies. There are also many medical doctors who are well informed on biological medicine and would find nothing objectionable in the programs outlined here.

How do you find these doctors?

Naturopathic physicians and chiropractors you can look up in the yellow pages of your telephone directory. For the biologically oriented medical doctors it would, perhaps, be better to ask the local chapter of the National Health Federation or ask in your favorite health food store for some names the owners might be familiar with. Because of the risk of pressure and malevolence from colleagues and medical organizations, the biologically oriented medical doctor would be reluctant to advertise his unorthodox affiliations or beliefs.

There are some clinics in the United States which use methods similar to those used in Swedish clinics, such as: Dr. Jensen's in Escondido, California; Dr. Max Warmbrand's Florida Spa in Orlando, Florida; Dr. H. Shelton's Health School in San Antonio, Texas; the Pawling Health Manor, Hyde Park, New York; and a few others.

It is my sincere hope that this book will stimulate awareness of biological medicine among practitioners of the healing arts and governmental health agencies. I am hopefully looking forward to a not too distant future when awakened interest on the part of arthritics, physicians, and health organizations will motivate them to conduct objective experiments with biological therapies in some of the major hospitals in the United States or Canada under 100 per cent scientific control. When such an experimental clinic becomes a reality, then American arthritis sufferers will be able to obtain biological treatments, as described in this book, right here in their own country under professional medical supervision. The united action of millions of people and aroused public opinion can break the frustrating chain of hopelessness, complacency, indifference, and medical prejudice and make the dream of every arthritic to be free from this agonizing disease a reality.

For the sake of all sufferers of arthritis, I hope this will happen soon.

Chapter 29

Recipes for Foods Named and Recommended in This Book

Below are recipes and directions for preparing dishes, dressings, beverages, juices, breads, etc. named and recommended in this book.

GREEN VEGETABLE SALAD

Use any available green or colored vegetables. Some of the "staples" recommended are: tomatoes, parsley, grated carrots, celery, cucumbers, any kind of head or leaf lettuce, green or red peppers, watercress, green onions, and avocado. But you may use "anything green," any of your favorites, such as cabbage, endive, radish, artichokes, celery root, red cabbage, beets, green peas, swiss chard, broccoli, cauliflower, kohlrabi, cantaloupe, watermelon, spinach, turnip tops, etc.

Wash vegetables carefully. Place green leaves, broken by hand, and other vegetables chopped, sliced, or shredded in a

big salad bowl. Add a couple of spoonfuls of your favorite vegetable oil (cold-pressed, available at health food stores), and
toss until everything is coated with oil. Then add the juice of
half a lemon, or two teaspoons of apple cider vinegar. Add your
favorite spices and herbs; paprika, anise, chili, watercress, mint,
basil, kelp, garlic, or whatever you have on hand (but no salt
or black and white pepper). Toss once more and serve immediately. This salad could be served separately, with cottage
cheese or some cooked vegetables, for example baked potatoes
or yams.

FRUIT SALAD À LA AIROLA

    1 bowl fresh fruits, organically grown if possible
    1 handful raw nuts and/or sunflower seeds
    3-4 soaked prunes or handful of raisins, unsulfured
    3 tbsp. cottage cheese, preferably homemade, unsalted
    1 tbsp. raw wheat germ
    1 tsp. wheat germ oil
    3 tbsp. yogurt
    2 tsp. natural, unpasteurized honey
    1 tsp fresh lemon juice

Wash all fruits carefully and dry. You may use any available
fruits and berries, but try to get at least three to four different
kinds. Peaches, grapes, pears, papaya, bananas, and fresh pineapple are particularly good to achieve a delightful bouquet of
rich, penetrating flavors. A variety of colors will make the salad
festive and attractive to the eye.

Chop or slice bigger fruits, but leave grapes and berries
whole. Place them in a big bowl and add prunes and nuts (nuts
and sunflower seeds could be crushed). Make a dressing with
one teaspoon of honey (or more if most of the fruits used are
sour), one teaspoon lemon juice, and two tablespoons of water.
Pour over the fruit, add wheat germ, and toss well. Mix cottage
cheese, yogurt, wheat germ oil, and one teaspoon of honey in a
separate cup until it is fairly smooth in texture and pour it on

top of the salad. Sprinkle with nuts and sunflower seeds. Serve at once.

This is not only a most delicious dish but it is the most nutritious and perfectly balanced, complete meal I know. It will supply you with high-grade proteins and all the essential vitamins, minerals, and enzymes you need for optimum health.

BIRCHER-BENNER APPLE MÜESLI

2 tbsp. old-fashioned oatmeal (not quick-cooking kind)
2 medium-sized apples
2 tbsp. wheat germ
2 tbsp. condensed milk or ordinary milk, fortified with
   1 tbsp. skim milk powder
2 tbsp. honey
½ lemon
2 tbsp. chopped nuts or sunflower seeds
1 tbsp. unsulfured raisins

Soak oatmeal overnight in four tablespoons of water. In the morning, add lemon juice and milk; mix well. Shred apples, unpeeled but well washed, into the mixture. Add honey, wheat germ, raisins, and nuts and stir. Serve at once, as it will lose in taste and food value if apples darken (oxidize).

This dish is a favorite at the famous Bircher-Benner biological clinic in Switzerland and is also very popular in health food restaurants in Europe.

GOLDEN OIL DRESSING

1 cup of any cold-pressed vegetable oil
1 tbsp. wheat germ oil
2 tsp. apple cider vinegar or lemon juice
2 tsp. honey
A touch of vegetable or sea salt, or kelp
Clove of garlic or your favorite natural
   herbs and spices (no pepper)

Place all ingredients in a glass jar and shake vigorously. By changing spices and herbs you can make an unlimited variety of different dressings using the same basic recipe.

AVOCADO DRESSING

1 avocado, ripe
2 tbsp. olive oil, or other cold-pressed vegetable oil
1 tsp. honey
2 tsp. apple cider vinegar or lemon juice

Cut avocado in half and remove the seed. Scoop out the pulp with a spoon and place in a blender. Add the other ingredients and run blender for a few seconds. If the mixture is too thick or doesn't cover the blades, add more oil. Delicious as a dressing for fresh vegetable or fruit salad.

CARROT JUICE

Take one pound of fresh carrots and wash well. Feed through the centrifugal juicer. (See health food stores for the models and prices.) This makes two glasses of a delicious and nutritious drink. This healthful juice is used extensively in biological clinics for treating arthritis.

CARROT-CELERY JUICE

Take equal amounts of carrots and celery and wash well. Feed through the juicer. Especially recommended in treatment of arthritis.

FRESH FRUIT JUICE

Excellent fresh juices could be made from the following fruits on a centrifugal juicer: apples, hard pears, and pineapples.

NUT-MILK

1 cup raw nuts or seeds
4 cups water
2-3 dates, 2 figs, or handful of raisins
1 tsp. honey, if dried fruits are not available

Any kind of raw nuts or seeds could be used, such as walnuts, almonds, filberts, peanuts, cashews, brazil nuts, sunflower seeds, sesame seeds, pumpkin seeds, chia seeds, etc. Note: chia seeds will make drink jell.

Place nuts and pitted dates, figs, or raisins in blender, add two cups of water, and run for about two minutes. Add remaining water, run for a few more seconds, and serve. It makes four servings.

BANANA MILK SHAKE (WITHOUT MILK)

1 cup crushed ice
1 ripe banana
1 cup raw nuts or seeds
1-2 dates, figs, or raisins
3 cups water

Place nuts and dates in blender, add two cups of water, and run for about two minutes. Add one cup of water and chopped banana and run for ten seconds. Add ice, run for ten more seconds, and serve. Add more water if needed. Makes four servings of highly nutritious drink.

HERB TEA

Use your favorite herbs. Health food stores carry a wide assortment of wholesome herb teas, such as: peppermint, white clover, camomile, fenugreek, alfalfa, rose hips, maté, etc.

Take one teaspoon of dried herbs for every cup of tea.

Bring water to a boil. Put herbs in the boiling water and immediately lift the pan from the heat, cover, and let stand ten to 15 minutes. Serve with natural, unpasteurized honey.

VEGETABLE BROTH

2 potatoes, chopped or sliced to approximately
  half inch pieces
1 cup carrots, shredded or sliced
1 cup celery chopped or shredded, leaves and all
1 cup any other available vegetables: beet tops,
  turnip tops, parsley, or a little of everything.
  However, broth could be made with only potatoes, carrots, and celery

Put all vegetables into a stainless steel utensil, add one and a
half quarts of water, cover and cook slowly for about a half
hour. Strain, cool to warm, and serve. If not used immediately
keep in refrigerator. Warm up before serving.

Vegetable broth is one of the standard beverages in all biological clinics in Sweden. Fasting patients always start the day
with a big mug of vegetable broth, a cleansing and alkalizing,
mineral-rich drink.

EXCELSIOR

1 cup of vegetable broth, as above
1 tbsp. whole flaxseed
1 tbsp. wheat bran

Soak flaxseed and wheat bran in vegetable broth overnight.
In the morning, warm up, stir well, and drink—seeds and all.
Do not chew the flaxseeds, drink them whole. Excelsior drink is
especially beneficial for patients with constipation problems. It
helps to restore normal peristaltic rhythm.

HOMEMADE YOGURT

Take a bottle of skim milk and heat it until hot-warm, but
do not boil it. Add two to three tablespoons of yogurt, which
can be bought in a grocery store or health shop. Stir it well.
Pour into a wide-mouthed thermos bottle. Cover and let it

stand overnight. In five to eight hours it will be solid and ready to serve. If you do not have a thermos jar, use an ordinary glass jar and place it in a pan of warm water over an electric burner switched on "warm" for four to five hours, then switch off until milk is solid.

Use two to three spoonfuls of your fresh, homemade yogurt as a culture for the next batch.

HOMEMADE COTTAGE CHEESE

First, make soured milk by adding two tablespoons of yogurt or cultured milk to each quart of lukewarm, unpasteurized milk. Keep in a warm place until it turns solid—12 to 24 hours.

Put bottle with soured milk in warm water, approximately 115° F., for one to two hours, until curdled. Place clean linen canvas over a dip strainer and pour curdled milk over it. Wait until all whey (clear yellowish liquid) has seeped through the strainer. What remains in the strainer is a wholesome and delicious homemade cottage cheese. If cheese is too hard, add a little sweet cream and stir.

POTATO CEREAL

1 big raw potato
2 tbsp. whole wheat flour
1 tbsp. wheat bran
1 tbsp. wheat germ
4 cups water

Heat water to boiling point. Mix flour and bran in pan and simmer for two to three minutes. Place a fine shredder over pan and quickly shred potato directly into pan. Stir vigorously and lift from the stove. Let it stand for a few minutes and serve hot with milk, butter, or cream; sprinkle wheat germ on top.

This is an alkaline and very nutritious cereal. It is used often in Swedish biological clinics, especially in diets for patients with arthritis.

MILLET CEREAL

1 cup hulled millet
4 cups water
½ tsp. honey
¼ cup powdered skim milk

Rinse millet in warm water and drain. Place in a pan of water mixed with powdered skim milk and heat mixture to boiling point. Then simmer for ten minutes, stirring occasionally to prevent sticking and burning. Remove from heat and let stand for a half hour or more. Serve with milk, honey, oil, or butter—or homemade applesauce! And treat yourself to the *most nutritious cereal in the world!*

MOLINO CEREAL

1 tbsp. coarse whole wheat flour
2 tbsp. wheat bran
2 tbsp. whole flaxseed
2-3 chopped figs
1 handful unsulfured raisins

Place all ingredients in pan with one cup of water and boil for five minutes, stirring occasionally to prevent burning. Serve immediately with fresh milk, a little honey, or applesauce.

WHOLE WHEAT BREAD
(Makes five 1 lb. loaves)

10 cups freshly ground whole wheat flour
4 cups warm water
2 packages dry yeast or 2 yeast cakes
2 tbsp. honey

Dissolve honey in cup of warm water. Sprinkle yeast over it and stir gently. Let mixture stand ten minutes. Pour the contents into a mixing pan, add remaining water and five cups of flour. Mix and beat well with an electric beater. Cover and let stand for 15 minutes. Add remaining flour and knead well. Dough should be moist but not sticky. Cover, place in warm area, and let it rise to double in size. Punch down and let it rise again. Knead and shape into loaves and put in greased pans. Let it rise once more until almost double in size. Bake 45 minutes at 350° F.

SOUR RYE BREAD
(Makes two 2 lb. loaves)

8 cups freshly ground whole rye flour
3 cups warm water
½ cup sourdough culture

Mix seven cups of flour with water and sourdough culture. Cover and let it stand in warm place overnight between 12 and 18 hours. Add remaining flour and mix well. Place in greased pans. Let it rise for approximately a half hour. Bake at 350° F., one hour or more, if needed. Always leave a half cup of dough as a culture for the next baking. Keep culture in a tight jar in your refrigerator. For the initial baking it would be necessary to obtain sourdough culture from a commercial bakery.

Index